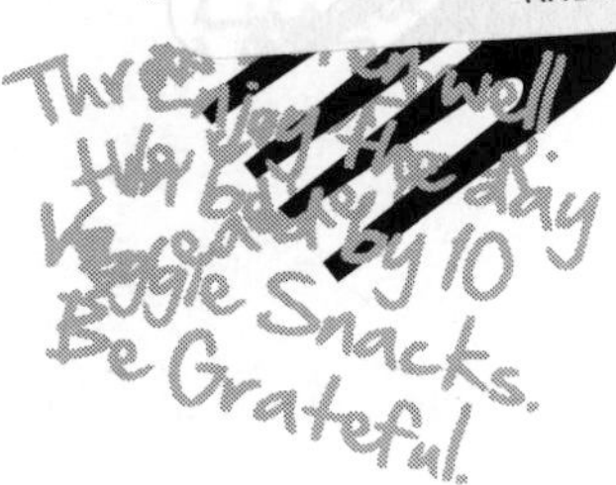

FULL PLATE

Nourishing your family's whole health in a busy world.

SARAH KOLMAN RN, MA

Full Plate: Nourishing Your Family's Whole Health in a Busy World by Sarah Kolman RN, MA.

Interior layout and cover design by Joanne Kophs Design. Contact Joanne at joanne@joannekophsdesign.com

ISBN: 978-1506145280

Printed in the United States of America

Table of Contents

THIS BOOK IS DEDICATED TO:

Jeremy, Cy, Joey, and Sam.

I hope to continue learning about health so that I can best support the happiness and wellness that you experience in your lives. I wish for you to live life with fullness and meaning for as long as you are meant to be here. Thank you for being such wonderful blessings in my life and giving me the gift of deep love and unconditional support. *My plate is full!*

Acknowledgements

It takes a village for this mama to write and publish a book. Thanks to the many people who have supported me in this journey. The following individuals provided exceptional support and guidance in this process and I can't thank them enough:

My warm-hearted, patient, and wise husband, *Jeremy Wilzbacher*, who sacrificed many nights helping me refine ideas and edit content. Your ongoing selflessness, encouragement, and love inspire me to live a meaningful life and make me feel capable of accomplishing great things. Thank you for helping me appreciate and love myself.

My mom and dad, *Fran and Al Kolman*, who have supported and loved me every step on my life's path. This process was no different. Thank you for your editing, feedback, encouragement, and willingness to care for the kids so I could crank this baby out. Oh yeah, and thank you for your ever-present, unconditional love—you keep my oxytocin flowing.

My sweet sissy, *Abbie Skoog*. Thank you for finding time in your full plate to read my entire manuscript and give me loving feedback about content and design and to engage in endless conversations that encouraged and inspired me in this process.

My mother-in-law, *Gini Wilzbacher*, whose gentle spirit and kind-heartedness always feel encouraging and loving. Thanks for proofreading and spending many tired evenings relaying silly errors.

Wendy Gebhart, my dear friend who sacrificed time with herself and her family to offer content feedback and suggestions. Your ability to provide gentle, loving, and clear-seeing guidance has had a foundational impact on my ability to complete this book. Thank you for being so instrumental in introducing me to whole health concepts and continually guiding my family's health.

Stefani Farris, writer and editor, was a breath of fresh air in the editing and refining phases of this process. Stefani is a talented writer, a gracious human being, and has been flexible with my evolving needs. Thank you for your commitment to my timelines despite a sick household, work deadlines, and your own family's full plate.

Graphic designer *Joanne Kophs* was amazingly patient with me during the cover design and interior layout process. You went above and beyond in developing the creative expression of the book. Thank you for providing extraordinary customer service and talent during all phases of this process. Joanne Kophs Design of Sammamish, Wash., comes highly recommended by me.

Thank you to *John Pierce* from Indianola, Wash., who helped edit references and guide me through the *Notes* process within my tight timeline.

Matt Copeland provided invaluable guidance and encouragement in the initial editing phases. Your ability to give loving and direct feedback is a skill that significantly impacted my ability to move forward in this process.

Susan Gose, a good friend, writer, and editor, was incredibly generous with her time and skillful feedback in the final editing phases. I appreciate your willingness to make corrections to the manuscript when your life is full with family, writing your own book, and editing others' books. Thank you for encouraging me through the last leg of the journey.

Denise Ackert inspired me with her willingness to read a stranger's manuscript and provide supportive and skillful feedback. Thank you for your selflessness and generosity.

The following individuals provided support, encouragement, and inspiration along the way; I thank you: Jagoe and Trey Warren, Tash and Gabe Harris, Stephanie Noll, Summer Nicklasson, Cristin Zimmer, Liz Grant, Emily Macdonald, Melissa Scherr, Soleiana Abernathy, Sarah Alme, Stephanie Addiss, Jeff Wilzbacher, Jess Rice, Lara and Chris Agnew, and Angie and Matt Flint.

Foreword

By Dr. Wendy Gebhart ND, MSOM

I've had the pleasure of reading this book in the midst of taking a year "off" from my busy life as a naturopathic medical doctor and mother of two young boys. It is heartening to think of how hard we as parents are working to provide the best life possible for our families and ourselves. As women, we are working outside the home more than we ever have before, yet we also have more activities available for our children, more demands placed on them in school, and more distraction by all things digital. Even if we have the information we need to live a more healthy life, even if we know what we need to do, we often end up prioritizing it below the many competing demands in our busy schedule. This was, in fact, one reason I chose to take a yearlong sabbatical with my family—to reprioritize *health* amidst our busy life.

I chose to make it a priority because every day in my office I see the consequences of prioritizing everything else above one's own health. I see patients, usually in their 50's, who have spent their lives caring for their children, working, buying beautiful things, taking wonderful vacations—and neglecting the very vehicle that makes all these things possible, their bodies. I know firsthand that planning for retirement will mean nothing for my husband and me if our bodies are disabled and diseased when we get there. The very conservative estimate by the Centers for Disease Control and Prevention suggests that more than 60 percent of the leading causes of death are preventable. This represents a shift in paradigm for even the generation I was raised in, which was taught that your chances for getting a particular disease are directly linked to your genes. There is now a whole field of science—*epigenetics*—that looks at how diet and lifestyle factors turn on or turn off your genes. The reality is that you do not have a predetermined disease destiny. You actually have the power and the responsibility to educate yourself to understand how you and your choices play a key role in health and healing. As parents, we can also make the greatest impact on the next generation by giving our children the tools and education to make health a top priority.

This is no small undertaking. I know that very few people are able to embark on a yearlong healing sabbatical. However, every person does have the ability to make small changes in her or his life. Small changes will in fact lead to lasting results if you take the time to educate yourself about the importance of and reasons for making these changes. In this book, Sarah provides you with very valuable information to educate yourself about the current understanding of disease and prevention. She also offers you concrete, useful tools that you can incorporate as you strive to improve your own health and the health of your family. Although I would recommend reading this book as a whole to gain a complete picture of the health information presented, each chapter shares many gems that will be valuable even if you can only read *Full Plate* in small bites.

I love Sarah's approach to primary and secondary foods. This perspective of balance between food as nourishment and all the other nourishing elements of our lives is a critical piece of health. I have seen many patients who have a "pristine" diet and are suffering with such stress from a job or relationship that they have as many or more symptoms of disease than the very stress-free couch potato with a loving relationship and fulfilling career. The time of picking apart symptoms and health is over, as we are each a whole interconnected system, and toxic relationships are no more or less damaging to our body and mind than toxic foods. Creating a balance between the food we put into our body and the nourishment we receive from relationships, career, sleep, and movement can help create an understanding of how valuable all our life choices are in our health.

Having firsthand experience from watching others move through their healing, I cannot emphasize enough: *health is an individual journey.* This reality is highlighted by the new information coming out every year regarding diet. I think we are finally understanding there is not a one-size-fits-all diet—or exercise program, sleep routine, or career path. One person's medicine is another's poison. Sarah highlights this individuality throughout her book, encouraging you to take the information and create a plan that works for you and your family. It is important to note that often when we are significantly "off" of our healing path, we might not even know how to make the healthiest choices for our body. If, for example, we are addicted to sugar or stress, there is a very real physiological process keeping us from making healthy choices. At these points in time, we need to follow the advice of health care professionals who have our healing goals in mind until we are able to connect clearly with the choices that are healthiest for ourselves and our families.

Full Plate is both a reminder to find what feeds you and nourish those things, and a guide to the many reasons that make this nourishment a priority. Sarah told me that her goal in writing this book was, first and foremost, to better understand the health choices she is making every day for her own family, but that she also hoped to share this information with those parents who might find interest or value in understanding a little more about health and healing but who feel their plate is too full to add one more thing. I think she has exceeded her goals by providing you with a household companion that will both educate you about and help you to implement whole health into your day-to-day life while still enjoying the fullness of your plate.

Dr. Wendy Gebhart ND, MSOM *is a Naturopathic Doctor with a Master of Science in Oriental Medicine. She is a mother of two and has enjoyed a private medical practice in Lander, Wyoming, for the last eight years.*

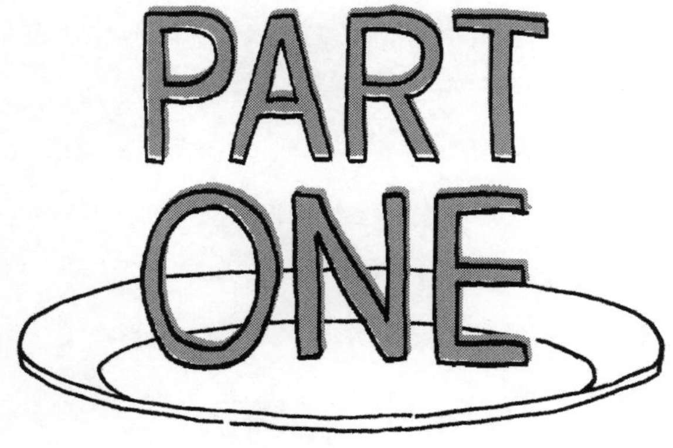

Introduction

1

Our Full Plate

I am one busy mama! I have three children, ages five and a half, four, and three. My husband travels two to three weeks out of every month, and in addition to parenting, I work part-time and go to school part-time. My days are full of hustling out the door on time, keeping my house and yard maintained, preparing three meals a day for my family, running to and from the kids' activities, school, and play dates, and trying to give my all to work and school. I'm surprised I even remember to feed the dog. In a typical day, I rarely sit down or stop moving. I am on the go! That goes for nighttime too. Just because the lights go out does not mean that my work as a mom is done for the night. My three-year-old has been waking up one to three times a night lately and the two older kids never fail to have a bathroom need or a nightmare—we often look like a three ring circus in the wee hours of the night! I have to make a very concerted effort to put attention towards "whole health" values because my life is set up for chaos, exhaustion, and ultimately an unhealthy lifestyle. I have a full plate.

Like me, the average American parent juggles a seemingly insurmountable number of tasks, activities, obligations, and stressors. Parents are stressed trying to balance work and family life, kids are involved in multiple extracurricular activities, on average we live farther from relatives and friends who traditionally have shared in childcare, and we live in a "connected" world that makes it hard to slip away from email, the telephone, the Internet, and television. Not to mention, the pressures from social media make it easy to constantly compare ourselves to others. Have you noticed that we live in a very competitive parenting world, where parents often feel pressure to give their children a "leg up?" We try to give our kids an edge by over-scheduling for soccer, swimming, basketball, ski lessons, dance class, etc. Even I feel the pressure to keep up with the Joneses. But there is not enough time in the day to juggle all of these demands. It is no wonder that parents complain about feeling tired, overwhelmed, inadequate, and defeated. We can't do it all, but we actually expect ourselves to do better than ever. Our plates are overflowing.

There is a hard truth to this reality. As we get busier something has to give. Our busy lives come with a cost. We are so distracted by our "activities" that we commonly sacrifice life balance and our health. It is not uncommon for families in our culture to habitually eat out (or in the car), carry high stressors, sleep poorly, and lack deep connection with each other as well as with our inner selves. Perhaps we are losing sight of the real advantage we can give our children.... health. In the scope of our children's entire lives, developing health nurturing habits will be a much more important factor for their future success than being a soccer star or the smartest kid in class. The focus that we put on work, activities, and tasks can distract our attention from core components of health. Science shows that our body's reaction to stress, loneliness, inactivity, poor sleep, and poor eating habits is directly related to illness and poor quality of life. Unfortunately, these are prevalent in our hectic lifestyles, contributing to why scientists have predicted that today's children will be the first generation in history to have a shorter life expectancy than their parents.[1]

You have probably heard, or noticed, that Americans are a pretty sick population. Obesity and diabetes are more common than ever and heart disease, dementia, ADD/ADHD, autoimmune diseases, cancer, and infectious diseases continue to rise—despite increased financial investment in healthcare. We try to manage disease through expensive treatments and pharmaceuticals, but we need to recognize that our real power to combat this epidemic lies in our ability to prevent and even cure disease through simple lifestyle changes.

More than ever, families are being called to reevaluate lifestyle priorities and values within their homes. There is no lack of nutrition and health advice available to us. Suggestions and advice are often overwhelming and contradicting. One expert tells you not to eat a particular food because it will make you fat and sick, while another expert tells you that you absolutely need it to flourish. There are quick fixes for weight loss and general health advice everywhere we look (few of which result in a sustainable lifestyle change). When was the last time you walked through a grocery store checkout line without some glamorous, half-naked woman offering you the key to health and a slim waistline? We are left to navigate a maze of conflicting and confusing information about how to live a healthy life. The information overload discourages most people from pursuing a healthy lifestyle, even when they have the desire and intention. As most of us can probably admit, the true path to health is much deeper than a fad diet. What you may not have realized is how widespread the factors are that impact our health. For example, did you know that our personal relationships can have just as much impact on our health as the food we eat? Did you know that how we feel about our work may be just as important as physical activity? Health is multi-faceted by nature. I refer to this comprehensive, integrative picture of health as "whole health," which is further explained and explored in the next chapter and will be the main theme that guides the content in this book. It is essential to look at our family's health from an interconnected approach.

The objective of addressing the stressors that create our "full plate" is not necessarily to strive for an "empty plate." Having a full plate is not inherently bad. In fact, I want my plate to be full—but in a meaningful way. My happiness and health come when my plate is full—full of healthy relationships, meaningful work, connection to my spirit, physical activity and rest, and nourishing foods. When my plate is full of experiences that feed my body, mind, and spirit, I feel healthy, happy, and complete. I am energized. On the other hand, when my plate is full of busyness and tasks that pull me away from connection, meaning, movement, and eating well, I feel distracted, disconnected, crabby, defensive, and, in general, lost. Our hectic, fast-paced lifestyles put us at great risk for the overextended full plate that disconnects and distracts us from what really matters—making us critically sick. The good news is that we have an opportunity to redirect our lifestyle to fill our plate with what fulfills us.

As you learn more about the various components of whole health in this book, you may feel pressured to "do more" or "add one more thing" in order to reach your health goals. I would encourage you to refrain from adding stress to your life by simply incorporating new tasks that you believe will magically make you healthy and happy. You will discover, rather, that when we begin to understand what fills our individual plates with meaning and happiness, we are naturally called to reprioritize tasks and activities. As we rearrange, substitute, and shift priorities, the most meaningful tasks begin to fill up the space in our lives. At the same time we begin to let go of the meaningless and harmful habits that have been consuming our attention and time. These refreshed perspectives and newly established priorities guide us and our families along a path leading to long and high quality lives. I offer this book as a guide to help you reflect on the behaviors and habits that might be depleting you, and to experiment with new practices and habits that will guide you to a nourished full plate.

2

Whole Health Philosophy

Health is more than just eating right and exercising. Throughout my career, one of the greatest truths I have witnessed is that health and happiness result not just from eating right and exercising, and not just from social and spiritual connection. After seeing so many transformations of health—from my time as a hospice nurse and a psychotherapist, as well as in my personal life—it is quite clear to me that health transformation occurs as a result of the integration of these and other factors. True health seems elusive when we focus only on one particular part of the health equation. We must give as much attention to our work, relationships, and spiritual connection as we do to food and exercise to truly optimize health. My studies at the Institute for Integrative Nutrition® have validated the larger truths that I have been experiencing since nursing school and have been integrating into my work as a nurse and counselor.

The primarily medical approach to health that I learned in nursing school focused on medical science, disease processes, physiology, and human anatomy. Although invaluable in establishing a foundation for understanding how the body functions and how disease manifests and progresses, in my early nursing career this medical focus always seemed to lack something fundamental. I enrolled in Naropa University's Masters in Contemplative Psychotherapy program in order to further expand my understanding of the complex mix of factors that affect and lead to health. Through mindfulness meditation practices, the program focused on psychology, human behavior, and the fundamental goodness within us all. Soon, I began to have "ah-ha" moments about what was missing in my nursing practice. We can't just nurse someone back to health medically; it is more complex than that. Achieving health is a broad pursuit, and at the same time unique to each person. Joshua Rosenthal, the founder of the Institute for Integrative Nutrition®, has established a structure within which these integrative components of health that I was discovering can be better understood. He breaks the elements of health into two categories: "primary food" and "secondary food."

Primary foods are fundamental parts of our lives that may even be of more "primary" importance than the food we eat when it comes to our health and wellness. To fully understand this concept, we need to think beyond the literal definition of food. We tend to think of food in a limited manner, as edible products that we ingest. Instead, the concept of primary food pushes us to think of food as substances, experiences, attitudes, and outlooks that nourish our body, mind, and spirit. We are fed by more than food alone. As I have experienced in my own career, a key aspect of health is balance and wellness within the following life arenas that Rosenthal identifies as primary food:

My Addition

1. *Meaningful Work*
2. *Healthy Relationships*
3. *Regular Physical Activity (and Adequate Sleep)*
4. *Connecting to Your Spirit*

Secondary foods are the physical, actual foods that we eat, the nourishment we put into our bodies. There is no one-size-fits-all food standard for everyone in the world. Indeed, as Rosenthal himself notes, "One person's medicine may be another person's poison" when it comes to food. Therefore, developing awareness of what eating strategies help each individual thrive is an important part of the equation. At the same time, despite the lack of any blanket recommendation for all individuals, there are overarching principles that guide us towards healthier eating habits that support the optimal functioning of our bodies. In later chapters, I will review how the standard American diet has significantly contributed to our current health crisis and how our families might be impacted if we don't follow some basic "real food" principles. Conversely, finding balance in primary and secondary foods in our own unique ways will enable us to live long, healthy, productive, and meaningful lives with our families.[1]

As I began to put together pieces of this puzzle in my own career, I slowly became aware of the thread that connected my insights on integrative health. Through attending nursing school, working as a hospice nurse, earning my degree in Contemplative Psychotherapy, and in my career ever since, I have come to believe that medical science and conventional "healthcare" are not currently set up to cultivate and inspire true health. Whole health depends upon the interconnectedness of meaningful work, healthy relationships, regular physical activity, adequate sleep, connecting to spirit, and consuming nourishing foods.

My highly valued nursing education took place at Marquette University, a Jesuit University that placed heavy emphasis on connecting and listening to inner spirit. In addition, community service was a core value at Marquette that taught me the importance of connecting with and serving others—regardless of career. I learned that helping others can be one of the keys to a fulfilled life. Then, while studying Contemplative Psychotherapy at Naropa, a Buddhist-based university with meditation practice at the core of its teachings, I began to see that when we are in alignment with ourselves and "still" inside we know best how to be with others. My Naropa education taught me that connection with myself is what fuels and inspires connection with others. I began to experience what connection did for my sense of well-being and health. Regular meditation was a requirement of the program, which led me to be with and know myself in a way that I had never done before. As I began to learn ways to help others see themselves more clearly in order to improve their relationships, careers, neurotic habits, and psychological ailments, I again discovered the complex nature of health, realizing that psychotherapy alone, as I had discovered with nursing, is rarely the sole solution. But when a variety of the elements of our life are nurtured and we find connection, discover meaning, know ourselves, eat nourishing foods, rest, and move our bodies, we do find health. In this book, I will share what I have learned in my education as well as through my professional experiences to help expand our understanding of whole health.

I have dedicated the bulk of my career to hospice nursing and have gained immeasurable lessons regarding health from the individuals with whom I have worked (including my own family members). Hospice is a service provided to people who have a prognosis of less than six months to live. It is aimed at helping them die in comfort, with dignity, and in the setting of their choice.

The patients I have worked with in hospice have been some of my greatest teachers about life and health, in two significant ways. First, my experience with hospice has given me insight into the fact that so many modern causes of death are the result of a lifetime of unhealthy habits and behaviors. I have seen how the evolution of the average American diet and lifestyle has led to widespread inflammation and disease. I have seen how miserable and painful cancer and chronic illness can be and see time and again that the majority of the population feels helpless to explain the causes of these illnesses. Most of us don't realize that the choices we make and the habits we develop affect us so greatly in our end. Others feel overwhelmed or powerless to change long ingrained lifestyle habits.

More importantly, however, my hospice patients have taught me inspiring lessons of life and love, and, perhaps ironically, they've taught me about health too. The vast majority of people entering hospice care have just transferred from the medical system, where they typically have spent the previous months or years focusing on aggressive medical treatments, fighting an illness or condition, and trying different strategies to "solve" a health problem. They have been fighting for quantity of life. But as people enter hospice there is a sense of slowing down. Patients are assigned a nurse, chaplain, social worker, doctor, nurse's aide, and volunteer. This team is designed to meet the psychological, spiritual, physical, and social needs of the patient, thus shifting the focus of care towards "primary food" in many ways. This team begins to ask the big questions, quality of life questions. As patients shift from a focus on quantity of life to a focus on quality of life, they tend to reprioritize what is really important to them. The best part of my job has been witnessing people transform and heal as they make decisions about how to spend their limited last days. Patients tend to focus on relationships, spirituality, and meaning. What has been truly awe-inspiring is to see how many patients actually begin to heal physically as they make these very "in-tune" decisions. The body is declining and the person is dying, but as he focuses on what matters, he experiences happiness, contentment, and, I would be bold enough to say, health. Witnessing these transformations has been revolutionary in the way that I think about health. Hospice is a great example of how tending to whole health improves our quality of life and extends our quantity of life. I have found that many hospice patients, suddenly comfortable for the first time in a long time, actually live longer than their prognosis. Studies have validated this observation, showing that when people receive hospice services early they actually live 25 percent longer than individuals who don't receive these service at all.[2] In addition to hospice care extending life, patients report feeling less depressed, less anxious, and more physically comfortable. One of the biggest insight hospice has provided me is that if nurturing our "primary foods" at the end of life can bring about transformational healing, imagine the impact we'd experience if we focused on these "whole health" influences throughout our lives.

My education at the Institute for Integrative Nutrition® is a perfect culmination of the insights that have enlightened my education and work, offering a framework for the truths that I have lived and felt in myself, and experienced with my patients and clients. As I am now fully engulfed in raising a family, I find that these truths from my career and education have parallel applications in family life. This is what I would like to share with you: first and foremost the powerful insights of "whole health" and how you can truly transform the way you experience the world. Additionally, I'd like to help you discover how to translate these realities into the hectic life that is parenting in the twenty-first century.

As we explore whole health it is important to keep in mind that health is a fluid concept. Unfortunately, we don't just reach a state of health and maintain that state perpetually. Health is a moving entity that ebbs and flows over time and is ever changing, as our bodies and lives change. Even our knowledge and understanding of what health means to us will change over time as we learn as individuals and as a society about healthy habits. This book provides many ways for you to integrate whole health concepts into your family's lifestyle if and when the time is appropriate for you and your family.

As you embark on this journey you and your family will likely encounter challenges. This is good and to be expected. Many of us clearly see that we have unhealthy lifestyle habits based on how we feel, look, and act, yet, there is no denying that change is difficult. Modifying lifestyle habits can be overwhelming and paralyzing. When we are used to a certain way of living and doing things it is hard to shift those habits, even if we know there is a better way. We are creatures of habit, are we not? At first modifying habits seems daunting, exhausting, and unattainable. However, once we become inspired by new insights, experience new ways of doing things, form new patterns, and gain tools we become better equipped to make those long-term changes. Fear and anxiety of the unknown are often our biggest hurdles in modifying lifestyle habits. Whether we take little steps toward our health goals or dive in headfirst with big shifts, we will notice that we eventually experience a new normal and our values naturally shift to support our new behaviors. I have a friend who was forced to change her diet significantly for major health reasons, and she was overwhelmed after learning about all the food she had to eliminate from her diet. Despite the challenge, health complications forced her to make the necessary modifications. She slowly incorporated the changes and with time shifted her values. She now makes decisions in her life based on her heightened values of healthy foods and self-care. Now that she has assimilated into her new lifestyle she doesn't feel overwhelmed by the changes. She feels empowered and confident in knowing what nurtures her health. Some people may relate to this dire need to change, while many others may not be driven to change by necessity. Often the greater challenge lies with the second group. The key to improving health is broadening our understanding of the factors that affect it, and targeting the simple, realistic, yet highly impactful lifestyle modifications that we can make.

The concept of whole health can actually make implementing changes more feasible as we begin to recognize how many options for improvement exist. We tend to focus on one or two items when we try to improve our lifestyle, usually diet and exercise. However, achieving health is much bigger, yet not necessarily more difficult, than just diet and exercise. Increasing our awareness of the array of lifestyle factors affecting health is important to achieve "whole health." The content in this book is designed to expand your framework of wellness and to encourage reflection and healthy modifications in areas that you identify as being important contributors to a potentially damaging or draining lifestyle. While I know we all strive for perfection, we can't be perfect when it comes to all of these components. In fact, perfection is discouraged. As important as the concepts are, take them lightly, allow yourself to play with them, and explore the ideas without having to *master* the whole health philosophy. In the end you will find that some or many of the concepts can easily fill your plate with health, without filling your plate with chaos.

☑ LIVE IT. MODEL IT. TEACH IT.

My "Live it. Model it. Teach it." philosophy is designed to provide you with three ways in which you can integrate whole health concepts into your own life and into your family system in a simple, practical manner. You will find this structure at the end of each chapter, starting in Part Two.

LIVE IT.

When we, as parents, live out a healthy lifestyle we gain the benefits of a healthy and happy life. Despite often feeling impossible, we deserve a high quality of life! Since I have become a mother I find that I often think about the health and happiness of my children significantly more than I think about my own. I tend to focus on my kids and mostly disregard my needs, especially when my husband is out of town and I am managing alone. Unfortunately putting myself last is not helpful or productive for anyone, including my children. When I am healthy and happy it benefits me, obviously, but my family is impacted positively as well. As parents, we owe it to ourselves and our families to prioritize a healthy and happy lifestyle for ourselves. We need to put attention on our own health for three important reasons:

1. To be more engaged and responsive in life, and less moody and reactive. Responsive, content, and energetic parenting is a more enjoyable experience to a family than tired, grumpy, and reactive parenting.

2. To have a high quality of life, with as little pain and illness as possible. Unhealthy lifestyle habits are scientifically shown to be the biggest contributor to chronic disease, poor quality of life, and premature death.

3. To set our bodies up for a long life of enjoyable experiences, including watching our children grow and evolve for as long as we are able.

MODEL IT.

When we live it, we are best able to model to the rest of our family what a healthy lifestyle looks like. Whole health will improve our relationships, our career satisfaction, our connection to spirit, how active we are, and what type of foods we put into our body. The most powerful teaching opportunity as a parent is to show our children what health looks like in all of these arenas through the way in which we live our lives.

TEACH IT.

Modeling is invaluable. But, passing down wisdom and information about health to our family is also an important piece of the puzzle. Many of us need to understand "why" before we can subscribe to a concept and feel confident in making decisions that are best for us. Surprisingly, our children also respond to the "why" more than many of us would expect. For example, in my family it is not uncommon for dinner conversation to involve a discussion about the magic of chlorophyll or how some nutrients make us strong and healthy and others might set our bodies up for illness and not feeling well. It is helpful to share with kids what we know about the benefits of the foods we eat and the things that we do, as well as the harm that certain foods or habits can have on our health. It is not helpful to put judgment on things that we try to avoid or do not value. For example, shaming others for eating fast food or having unhealthy lunches at school is not helpful. It is best to concentrate on the knowledge that we have and the reasons for which we make our decisions. Our goal is for our children to have information and knowledge in order to make informed decisions for themselves, not to condemn and judge others for their choices.

This book will provide tools and knowledge for you to live a healthy lifestyle, model it to your family, and teach information, insight, and rationale so that your family can be informed and empowered to make their own decisions about their health choices. The "whole health" perspective outlined in this book will enable you to look at many aspects of your life and decide what areas you want to put attention towards in order to enhance your health and happiness. Implementing lifestyle modifications that may at first seem overwhelming and difficult will become easier than you expect.

3

Inflammation Affects All Aspects of Our Health

Cellular inflammation in the body is now thought to be at the root of the most disabling and common illnesses in modern society, and is caused and sustained by many of our habitual lifestyle practices.[1] Understanding the impact of inflammation is an essential link to appreciate the connection between our lifestyle factors and disease and illness, and therefore the link between health and the wide-ranging strategies aimed at decreasing inflammation.

Inflammation is the body's attempt to protect itself. The purpose of inflammation is to remove harmful substances, like damaged cells, irritants, or pathogens, and to initiate the healing process. When something harmful or irritating affects a part of our body, there is a biological response to try to remove it. This process brings about the signs and symptoms of inflammation: local redness, heat, swelling, and pain in the affected area of the body. It is the body's natural healing response. Acute, short-term inflammation is the body's way of healing itself by bringing nourishment and immune activity to a site of injury or infection. Infections, wounds, and tissue damage would not heal without inflammation. Instead, tissue would become more and more damaged. Inflammation is our body's way of dealing with acute, short-term attacks on the body. However, when inflammation is stimulated on a prolonged or chronic basis, when no threat is present, its effects on the body become more complicated. The constant production of immune cells resulting from this effect no longer serves a specific purpose, and can result in tissue damage and illness. This is called chronic inflammation, and it can be caused by stress, poor diet, exposure to toxins, poor sleep habits, sedentary lifestyle, and loneliness (yes, even loneliness), to name a few.[2]

Chronic inflammation is more and more becoming recognized as the root cause of many serious illnesses, including heart disease, diabetes, ADD/ADHD, stroke, obesity, migraines, thyroid disease, many cancers, Alzheimer's disease, asthma, allergies, and depression.[3] Because inflammation manifests as so many types of chronic and life-threatening illnesses, many experts are now realizing that chronic inflammation is essentially the leading cause of death in the United States.[4]

Dr. Andrew Weil is a medical doctor, naturopath, teacher, and author on holistic health and is well known for establishing the field of integrative medicine. Weil has identified many of the connections between inflammation and disease, and frequently recommends an anti-inflammatory diet (similar to the Mediterranean diet) and lifestyle changes in order to combat them. Weil explains that coronary heart disease begins as inflammation in the arteries and Alzheimer's disease begins as inflammation in the brain (which, from his perspective, is why ibuprofen, an anti-inflammatory, has a preventative affect against Alzheimer's disease). He also notes that India—a country that traditionally uses large amounts of turmeric (one of the most potent natural anti-inflammatory substances) in their cooking—also has one of the lowest rates of Alzheimer's disease in the world. In his opinion, even links between inflammation and cancer are beginning to make sense. For example, anything that is pro-inflammatory causes cells to divide more frequently, which results in an increase in malignant replication—in other words, cancer. Similarly, he claims that aspirin's powerful anticancer affect is due to its anti-inflammatory properties. The good news is that if many chronic diseases have a common root (inflammation), then there may also be a common solution (a hint, it is not popping aspirin on a daily basis). We often want quick fixes and medications in our society in order to make us well. Masking symptoms with medications, such as anti-inflammatory drugs, can cause other illness-related issues from the side effects (some of which are life-threatening). In addition, masking the symptoms in a way gives us permission to continue living the lifestyle that likely caused the problem in the first place. Instead, we can treat the underlying root cause of the problem by understanding the ways in which we create cellular inflammation in our bodies and consequently reverse that process through lifestyle changes. Anything we can do to keep inflammation at bay (I will share many of them) will help us prevent disease, live longer, and feel healthier.[5]

Unfortunately, chronic inflammation itself typically does not produce noticeable symptoms until actual loss of function occurs somewhere in the body. Chronic inflammation often manifests at imperceptible levels, often silently damaging our tissue over an extended period of time. This process can go on for years without being noticed, until seemingly out of nowhere we are diagnosed with a serious condition or disease. Chronic illnesses occur often after a lifetime of inflammatory damage.[6] The slow onset of disease is problematic in that people often do not make the connection between their ongoing poor health habits and low grade symptoms or the condition that "appeared out of nowhere." It is hard to see our bad habits as problematic if we don't notice detrimental damage until it's too late. In some ways it's like maintaining a car. If we let the little problems go unnoticed, the car will eventually develop bigger problems and peter out, not lasting as long as it could have if it had been cared for and maintained. My dad always says, "If you take care of your machines, your machines will take care of you." Similarly, if we take care of our body, our body will take care of us. By maintaining and fine tuning health our body will run smoothly and lead to a high-mileage life. And one of the most important ways to maintain health is to manage cellular inflammation.

When I was a freshman in college, I regularly suffered from body aches and pains as well as general fatigue. After perplexing many doctors, I was finally diagnosed with Fibromyalgia. Fibromyalgia is a common diagnosis given to people who have generalized pain of unknown origin. I was put on muscle relaxers to help with the daily discomforts I experienced. The muscle relaxers did a great job of making me want to sleep much of the day and negatively affecting my engagement in school. I accepted the Fibromyalgia diagnosis and treatment for several years. Later, motivated by a book I read about the harmful effects of sugar and processed foods, I eliminated refined sugars and highly processed foods from my diet. When I made these changes, my daily aches and pains vanished. It turns out that I did not have Fibromyalgia and most definitely did not need muscle relaxers. The aches and pains I was experiencing were the result of the inflammation my body was experiencing from the sugar and processed foods that I was eating every day. To this day when I eat sugar or processed foods, I immediately feel my body ache—an instantaneous reminder of the inflammation that arises when I eat such foods. What I feel as discomfort might be acute inflammation in my body if it is a one time occurrence; however it becomes chronic inflammation when I continue to eat those foods, causing debilitating, constant inflammation in my body. Not everybody feels a direct response to harmful foods, like I do with sugar and processed foods, but that doesn't mean that chronic inflammation isn't silently taking place, at unperceivable levels in the body.

Our diet is an important part of keeping chronic inflammation at bay. It is important to realize that dietary components can either trigger or prevent inflammation from taking root in our bodies.[6] Certain foods, such as trans-fats and sugars, can be pro-inflammatory, meaning they cause and support inflammation in the body. And excess omega-6 fatty acids increase inflammation, while omega-3 fatty acids decrease inflammation.[7] Americans typically consume high amounts of omega-6 fatty acids, tipping the scale towards inflammation. We will later discover how these and other foods influence the inflammatory process and that we are able to use food to contain inflammation and reduce long-term risk of disease.

It may be obvious that our diets could impact chronic inflammation, but diet is not the only factor. Unhealthy lifestyle habits outlined in the next four chapters can also contribute to chronic inflammation. We will explore how the lifestyle choices that we make really do impact inflammation in our bodies—and have other related health ramifications, as well. The good news is that there are practical ways we can decrease cellular inflammation and improve our health through work, relationships, physical activity, rest, and connecting to ourselves in a deep way. We get to use the many opportunities in our busy day to turn negative, draining, disease-causing habits into practices of nourishment, meaning, and connection for ourselves and the whole family.

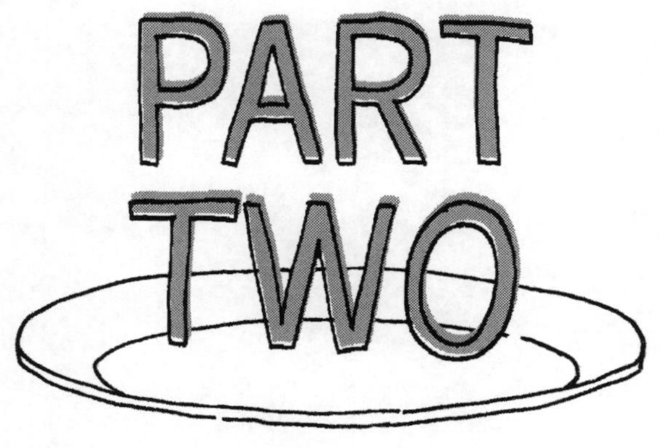

Primary Food

4

Meaningful Work

The level of engagement we have in our work and the meaning that work holds for us impacts our health on a very real level. Our work or occupation typically takes up more than half of our waking hours. Often it consumes significantly more time when you consider the time we spend thinking or worrying about obligations, deadlines, or projects during our non-work hours. Therefore, when our work is a source of stress, as it can be for many of us, we may spend the majority of our week in a stressed state. If our work is not meaningful to us we may spend this work time disengaged, simply tolerating a livelihood that does not fill us. The negative consequences of these experiences on our body are significant. In addition to causing poor quality of life they literally cause illness.

When we speak of work in this regard we refer to more than the typical job that some of us perform for eight hours a day, five days a week. Our "work" includes all alternate versions of occupations, vocations, or regular responsibilities. Many of us dedicate our time to managing our homes, yards, kids' activities, and family finances. Others work their land as farmers and ranchers. Some do a mixture of formal work and managing a home. Whatever you regularly dedicate your time to that supports the lifestyle that you and your family enjoy is your work. When reading this chapter and reflecting on your own level of "work" satisfaction and stress, think outside of the box and apply the concepts and tools to all of the activities that you perform on a regular basis.

Find Work You Love or Love the Work You Have

It is no surprise that happiness does not come from money or the "right job." Yet it is not uncommon for many of us to get lured into occupations that provide nothing more than a paycheck and the security of having a "responsible" career. Our work may end up void of meaning and in some cases force us into a semi-numb state because we are not inspired or fulfilled by what we do. Worse yet, many people spend years in careers that are completely opposed to what they feel is their higher purpose in life. But this is our one precious life! Bringing congruity to who we are and what we do in this world has a big impact on our satisfaction in life and, as we will discuss, our overall health.

In his book, *A Hidden Wholeness: The Journey Toward an Undivided Life*, Parker Palmer highlights the importance of living a life "undivided," a life that merges our soul with our role. Palmer states that because we are "afraid that our inner light will be extinguished or our inner darkness exposed, we hide our true identity from each other. In the process, we become separated from our own souls. We end up living divided lives, so far removed from the truth we hold within that we cannot know the integrity that comes from being what you are."[1] I relate to Palmer's claim. It is vulnerable and scary to know what my deepest desires are and to go out and live them. What if I fail? What if I am truly seen and people don't accept me? What if someone judges me for what I do? On the flip side, I feel safe having a job that allows me to hide behind a role that is separate from who I am deep inside. If I fail or if I am judged, the stakes are not as high because I am actually hiding from my true essence, my true vulnerability. Brene Brown has written numerous books and has been recognized nationally for her work on the power of vulnerability. She claims that it takes tremendous courage to be vulnerable and to completely show up in life and in relationship, but that when we do we reap priceless rewards through the enhanced quality we find in both.

I believe that we all really want to be passionate and engaged in the work that we do. We want our true selves to be in alignment with our careers and the lives that we lead. Unfortunately, many forces make the "divided life" the easier path. It is easier to keep a job in the career that you chose when you were eighteen, for which most of us are still paying student loans fifteen years later. We may even feel an internalized obligation to stay in a job. It can be easier to stay in a good paying job that demands long hours and tears at the soul simply because there is security in a paycheck, responsibilities at home, and convenience in familiarity. It is often difficult to know what the "perfect" job is, so we might hide behind the face of "not knowing," out of fear of taking a chance, risking failure, or being fully seen.

In her final episode of the *Oprah Winfrey Show*, Oprah said, "Live from the heart of yourself. You have to make a living, I understand that. But, you have to know what sparks the light in you so that you, in your own way, can illuminate the world."[2] When our work is in alignment with our passion or with what we know to be in sync with our essence, we are unstoppable, creative, and most productive. The world, and we, reap the benefits. But it's not always easy to know what "sparks the light" in us. Sometimes simply paying attention to what we *don't* want to do can lead us into figuring out what we *do* want to do. We usually can feel when something isn't the right fit for us. However, we can be distracted from this feeling by blindly doing the work that we are familiar with or believing that we don't have control over what we do for work, that we have no choice. We find reasons to avoid listening to our inner self telling us that something isn't working. Yet, it is important that we listen to our truth. We may feel confused between what the world is saying to us versus what our inner selves are saying to us. Theologian and activist Howard Thurman wisely said, "Don't ask what the world needs. Ask what makes you come alive, and go do it. Because what the world needs is people who have come alive."[3] We must ask ourselves what it is that we are drawn to, what makes us come alive. So go ahead and ask yourself. In my heart, is the work I am doing making me come alive?

Answering this question honestly for ourselves gives us the opportunity to experience this one life we have in the most connected, fulfilling, and healthy way possible. Try answering this question for yourself with a loved one. You may find that speaking out loud makes it hard to stick with your same old stories ("I have no choice in what I do." "My family needs me to do this work." "I have to do this because this is what I invested my college education in." Or, "This is all I know how to do."). These excuses don't hold up when held up to the light (or your trusted friend's ear). Recently, I was faced with listening to my inner voice encouraging me to make changes in my career. I was being pulled between my work as a hospice nurse and my role as a mother. Especially when my husband was traveling, I felt like the juggling of all of my roles was causing stress, disconnectedness with my family, and complete exhaustion. I knew that resigning or significantly cutting my hours was best for me. However, the reality of considering financial stressors was a big concern in making the leap. I talked it through with my friends and husband endlessly, and they all reflected to me that it was clear that I knew what I needed and reassured me that the financial implications were workable. I ended up cutting my hours back significantly and scheduled more time in my home to manage housework and slowdown in an attempt to diminish stressors and take better care of myself. Through tweaking our budget, the financial adjustments have been workable, and I am grateful that I had the courage to trust my inner voice directing me towards those needed changes. I can see how easy it is to convince ourselves that big, and sometimes scary, changes are not practical or realistic. I am glad that I didn't buy into the stories my mind created.

Some of us have legitimate restrictions on the choices and opportunities available to us due to education, local job markets, immigration status, and other factors. But many of us have mental blocks that prevent us from believing we have other options. Whether a CEO of a large corporation or a dishwasher in a restaurant, our occupation can either connect us to ourselves and what we see as our purpose in life, or it can drain us and force us to live with the divided self. The first step is to ask yourself: "In my heart, am I doing what I am meant to be doing, what makes me come alive?" As we honestly answer that first question a vision of our purpose in life begins to develop. The second step is then to creatively examine what can move your career to be more in line with your soul's calling in life.

I'm not suggesting that you need to leave your career. The goal is to find work you love, or learn how to love the work you have. Many of us don't have to leave our job in order to have a fulfilling career. There are many ways to find gratification and connect our calling to our job. You may stay in your same career but need to move to a different company, a different boss, or simply change your perspective or attitude about what you want to get out of your work. For some, it's a matter of establishing boundaries and priorities, or improving communication with supervisors or co-workers. If you give yourself some space and are honest with yourself you will know whether you need to change careers, tweak some aspect of your current situation, or change nothing at all. Simply try not to let fear get in the way of doing what it is you truly want to do.

As parents we are not the only ones who can get caught up in the pressures of doing things for the wrong reasons. Finding work we love and loving the work we have also applies to our children, even though they don't technically have a career. The "work" of a child comes in the form of school, extracurricular activities, and general play. Helping our children be in touch with what nourishes them now will establish the patterns and habits that they carry into adulthood. As a parent of three young children living in a very active community where kids are often involved in two, three, four, or more activities at a time, I see how easy it could be for children to learn to do what is expected of them instead of doing what suits their passions and interests. Whether they feel expectations to be on the advanced soccer team, in competitive swimming, a straight-A student, or simply be on the same team as their best friends, kids feel pressure regularly. Left unchecked these multiple demands on our children can teach them to be motivated by external expectations set by teachers, parents, coaches, or friends, rather than to look within to discover what drives them. It is important that children are learning how to merge their inner spirit with what they choose to spend their time doing. If a child is overwhelmed mentally and perpetually exhausted from participating in multiple activities (or even just one "wrong" one) perhaps some activities should be reconsidered. If children don't thrive in school we can help them work through challenges and connect what they are motivated by to what the school experience has to offer. If we can't teach children the skill of self-awareness and knowing how to listen to their inner drives, they will continue into their careers with the same crutches and challenges as many of us, ultimately affecting both their career satisfaction and their physical health. We want to teach our children the importance of doing what they love and loving what they do, an invaluable lesson that will frame their happiness throughout their lives.

Chronic Stress

Stress can and does occur for most of us in many areas of life, but it is particularly important to talk about stress when reflecting on work. Americans are known for putting pressure on ourselves at work. We place high demands on ourselves, as well as on others, in the work environment. We can be perfectionists, work long hours, try to meet unreasonable deadlines, and do the work of others because we think we can do it better. When these stress-inducing behaviors become day-to-day activities, they can lead to chronic stress. The American Psychological Association has found that about 25 percent of Americans experience high levels of stress (rating their stress level as eight or more on a ten-point scale), while another 50 percent report moderate levels of stress (a score of four to seven).[4] That means 75 percent of Americans report moderate to high levels of chronic stress. Many of us recognize and even accept continuous levels of stress as part of our lives, but we may not fully appreciate the fact that chronic stress has serious implications for the health of our bodies.

Stress is your body's response to any real or imagined threat. It is a natural response and can be advantageous when it helps protect us from harm. If we are being chased by a dog our sympathetic nervous system kicks in with a "fight or flight" response. This is an evolutionary survival function, enabling people and other animals to react quickly to life-threatening situations. The cascade of hormonal changes and physiological responses helps someone to fight the threat off or flee to safety. A stressful incident can trigger physiological changes like increased heart rate, rapid breathing, muscle tension, and sweating. Ideally, these physiological responses cease once you have climbed the tree and escaped the chasing dog. Unfortunately, the body can overreact to stressors that are not life-threatening, such as work stress, family difficulties, or health challenges. Over time, this stress becomes chronic. So when we feel continuously overwhelmed or overworked, we never escape the dog and our body never gets a chance to regain its natural state of relaxation. This overexposure to stress can disrupt almost all of our body's processes. A key component of "whole health," then, is to neutralize stress in order to protect our bodies.

The main hormone excreted when we experience stress is called cortisol. The human body has two adrenal glands, one on top of each kidney. These glands secrete hormones—including cortisol—that act as "chemical messengers." Under the fight or flight response, though, cortisol serves us by providing a quick burst of energy, lowers sensitivity to pain, and improves memory. Under evolutionary survival conditions, this short term response would almost always be followed by a period of no stress—you kill the lion and the danger disappears—during which your body would return to normal functioning. When we are faced with chronic stresses, however, we lack the normal relaxation periods that bring our body functions back to normal. In this "non-normal" state, the typically helpful cortisol actually begins to have harmful effects on our body. Chronic stress, and the consistent release of cortisol, causes many physical and psychological problems. For one, excess cortisol is toxic to nerve cells in the hippocampus, the part of the brain that controls memory and emotion, impacting our ability to recall memories and maintain stable emotions.[5] Cortisol-related changes in the brain have been shown to contribute to anxiety, depression, and addiction. Repeated activation of cortisol takes a toll on the physical body, as well. Research suggests that chronic stress contributes to heart disease, digestive problems, decreased immune functioning, intestinal bacterial imbalance, poor metabolism, interrupted sleep, increased insulin, relationship conflicts, and weight gain (in particular storing fat around the midsection), even if you don't eat more. Cortisol has also been shown to have an inflammatory affect in the body, which means that chronic stress contributes to chronic inflammation—resulting in disease and illness.[6] The impacts of stress are powerful enough to negate even a "perfect" diet. It affects our bodily systems widely and profoundly.

When I experience high levels of stress it is usually obvious to me, even in the moment. What is more challenging to see is what can be a lower level, more subtle stress that is less recognizable. I have realized that this less obvious—but almost always present—type of stress is my Achilles heel in life. When I slow down and notice my shallow breathing, tight body, and edgy state of mind, I clearly see the amount of chronic stress I unknowingly carry. As I work to manage all of life's responsibilities, at work and at home, I maintain a subtle state of stress and anxiety. This state feels normal to me—because it is my normal. I have come to realize that my body and mind rarely regain their natural state of relaxation. I'm learning how damaging this chronic state is for my overall health, and it requires pretty focused attention to shift my "normal" state into one that is more relaxed.

Physical activity, meditation, yoga, relaxation, a hot bath, listening to music, focusing on something of interest, and practicing gratitude can be helpful stress relievers of which you may be familiar. Incorporating any of these or other similar practices into our routine moves us one step closer to a lowered level of stress. Interestingly, we have another stress relieving tool right under our nose that is even more powerful than some of these well-known strategies. Believe it or not, breathing is one of the best tools for stress reduction. By changing the way we breathe in any given moment, we literally change our physiological state. We can interrupt the cascade of hormones that are released following the initiation of the "fight or flight" response. Breathing is one of the most central and powerful functions of the human body. It is one of only a few bodily functions that we can perform both voluntarily and involuntarily, thereby crossing a barrier that is not possible for most of the body. By practicing particular breathing techniques we have the ability to influence the autonomic nervous system (which stimulates the fight or flight response). In other words, voluntarily imposing rhythms on the breath gradually induces those rhythms in the involuntary nervous system, positively impacting circulation, digestion, and other important functions of the body. According to Dr. Andrew Weil, a basic rule for breathing practice is to try to make your breaths deeper, slower, and more regular. To deepen your breathing practice, continue to exhale beyond your normal breathing sequence. By squeezing more air out you will automatically breathe more in. Weil recommends the following breathing technique which he calls the "4-7-8 Breath" as a way to positively change your breathing rhythms and begin to lower stress levels:

4-7-8 BREATH

1. Forcefully exhale, making a wind noise.
2. Breathe in through your nose for 4 seconds,
3. Hold your breath for 7 seconds.
4. Release air through your mouth for 8 seconds.
5. Repeat four times at least twice daily.

According to Weil, this breathing technique is the most powerful anti-anxiety intervention you have available to you. You can't be upset or anxious and perform this exercise at the same time. In addition to practicing this breathing technique religiously twice daily, Weil recommends doing it during stressful moments in your day (working on overwhelming projects, listening to screaming kids, dealing with relationship conflict) in order to neutralize stress on the spot. He claims it can literally change the autonomic nervous system (the "fight or flight" response center). Weil suggests that if you follow this technique twice daily for six to eight weeks, you will find notable changes in your mental and physical health. Weil's example is just one breathing technique that you can try; there are many styles and instructions for conscious and controlled breathing. I suggest trying several until you find one that works best for you and your lifestyle.[7]

Soul-Centered Self-Care

In order to sustain our work and manage the stressors that come with it, it is worth considering ways in which we take care of ourselves and prevent burnout. I believe that self-care is a cornerstone of wellness and balance. That said, I also find self-care to be incredibly hard to implement as a mother tending to a busy household. I have struggled with self-care for most of my life. But I've found that when I neglect it, the repercussions come out in ugly ways. I once felt so overwhelmed and stressed that I'd finally had it: I told my husband I was going to check into a hotel for the night to just escape it all. Worse was the time that I felt just shy of a mental breakdown and threatened to fly as far across the country as I could to get away from my family and my life. And does throwing a breakfast sausage across the kitchen and telling my kids that they were little __________ (fill in the blank with a word that I can't bring myself to share with the world) count as an actual mental breakdown? The accumulation of exhaustion and lack of self-care seems to always come back to haunt us. Therefore, I'm trying to learn to implement continuous and regular self-care to avoid these explosions. Why does such a nice, inviting concept as "care for self" seem so daunting and why do I so frequently push it to the bottom of my list of priorities?

I have come to learn that I have misunderstood the concept of self-care, assuming that self-care meant carving time out of my busy day to journal, exercise, get a massage, garden, meditate, and eat healthy foods. Self-care was one more thing I *had* to do. And I didn't always want to do those things. I wasn't inspired to do self-care as I imagined it, so it was the first thing to fall off of my to-do list.

Broadening my understanding of self-care helped me improve my relationship with it. Marilena Minnucci, a health coach and author, talks about "soul-centered self-care." She says that soul-centered self-care is a practice that is in alignment with who we are and is not based on "shoulds" and "should nots." It is heart-centered and not head-centered, and it builds internal resilience and strength. At the core of this type of self-care is understanding who we are and what we desire. Caring for our self needs to be a joy, not an obligation.

Self-care turns into self-love when we honor our day and our life with things that fill our cup. It is a reflection of the love we have for ourselves because we know what makes us smile, breathe, and relax. This type of self-care is something we need to discover for ourselves through experimentation. It is not easily found from online advice, in a book, or from another person. In soul-centered self-care, we are in charge of whatever it is that fills us.

When we have a practice of regular self-care, our personal, professional, and family lives will more naturally fall into balance. Look at everything in life through the lens of self-care. We must ask ourselves: "What gives me energy, and what drains my energy?" If we can drop things that aren't "filling our plates," it is worth considering. If we can't drop things because they are a necessary part of life, then we should find ways to make them enjoyable. For instance, doing the dishes used to be a cause for stress in my life, but dirty dishes are an unavoidable part of life. I can't just stop doing the dishes. I needed to find ways to make the task enjoyable. I now wash all of the dishes before dinner even begins, so that when dinner is done I only have a small handful to do. The small amount of dishes left after dinner actually excites me (like a silly game with myself) because the task is now completely manageable and simple, rather than overwhelming. Or, when cooking dinner feels like a task, I may drink a glass of wine or put on music while I cook (or both!), and it becomes a more pleasurable event. During one period when we were being tortured by our second child's daily five o'clock wake-ups, my husband started simply waking up and taking him for a run in the stroller. He was able to transform an *energy drain* into an *energy fill*. The goal is to identify sources of stress and transform them into practices of self-care in a way that works for you. The process helps us identify what gives us ease and brings us closer to who we are.

As parents, we experience natural stumbling blocks to maintaining self-care. Although attending to the formation of a family is rewarding work, we tend to neglect ourselves and become distracted from honoring that which nurtures us. We also tend to focus on the million and one things that we have to get done in our week. The very last thing on our list would be doing something to pamper ourselves. Be aware not to let busyness validate you as a person and pull you away from meeting your own needs. At the end of the day we have to fill our plates with meaning and care. If we don't, we ultimately have less and less to give to our family.

Striving for perfection in self-care can be a trap. We may not even attempt to meet our own needs because we believe we won't be able to do it right. Perfectionism inhibits healthy self-care because we usually set unreachable expectations. Taking care of yourself does not have to mean transforming your lifestyle, becoming an athlete, or adding additional tasks to your already busy life. Often, all that is needed is to recognize what drains you, and explore how to transform that experience into something that can fill you. You may not know the answer right away. In this process there is no failure, there is only learning. Try to let go of the fear of failure, as it is often what makes the experience stressful. If you try something new and it doesn't remove the "drain," then try something else. Eventually we will find some simple solutions that truly do transform energy drains into energy sources. The more we identify things that drain us, the more we will begin to shed those elements from our life.[8]

☑ LIVE IT. MODEL IT. TEACH IT.

LIVE IT.

- ☐ Find the work you love and love the work you do. Ask yourself if your work is in alignment with your higher purpose in life. Dare to find work that best suits your passions and interest.

- ☐ Identify stressors at work, and in other areas of life. Focus on the true source of that stress. Think of things that will lessen that stress, and practice conscious breathing exercises to interrupt stressful experiences.

- ☐ Experiment with Weil's "4-7-8 Breath" in your daily routine twice a day.

- [ ] Reflect on what elements in life fill you and what elements drain you.

- [ ] Find soul-centered self-care activities to take care of yourself so you don't burn out. Integrate self-care into the activities that you already do throughout your day, especially activities that are typically draining. When we value taking care of ourselves we start interacting with our family (and others in the world) differently. This is a priceless gift that we give our family.

- [ ] Schedule regular time in your calendar for activities that you love and that fill you up. Use this time to reflect, relax, and recharge.

MODEL IT.

- [ ] Doing what we love and loving what we do shows our children that life is not about meeting the expectations that others have for us. Life is about listening to our inner wisdom, knowing what moves us, and not always letting external expectations guide our engagement in life.

- [ ] We as parents have a powerful opportunity to demonstrate to our kids what it means to relax, enjoy life, and love ourselves. If they watch us take care of ourselves they will learn what it looks like to practice self-care and have the skills to implement it in their own lives. If they watch us work non-stop and spread ourselves thin with commitments they will learn that those are life values, and repeat the harmful patterns they observe.

TEACH IT.

- [ ] Help your children figure out what extra-curricular activities really fill their emotional and spiritual plates. Offer support and guidance to a child that may not be interested in some of the activities in which he or she is involved.

- [ ] Have open discussions about what is going well and not so well in your children's lives, and help them decipher what they can remove from their full plates, the activities that do not fill them, and how they can improve their experience with the things that can't be removed.

- [ ] Inquire about what family members enjoy doing and help them carve out time on a daily basis to rest, enjoy life, and do what they love.

- [ ] Teach your children about activities and practices that will help them manage stress, including deep breathing exercises like "4-7-8 Breath."

- [ ] Teach your family about soul-centered self-care and the importance of tending to those activities that bring us joy and relaxation.

5

Healthy Relationships

The health of our relationships influences so many aspects of our lives. Have you ever had an argument with someone that made you feel grumpy and agitated for the rest of the day? Or, maybe you have been in conflict with your partner for a couple of weeks and you find yourself thinking about it obsessively. You may even notice that you have a headache, are sleeping poorly, and indulging in your favorite flavor of ice cream (or wine). Some of us feel the impact of our relationships viscerally and clearly. When I am not in a good relationship with my husband or kids, I feel like I am on fire inside and everything that I do seems to be affected. It is truly an awful feeling. For others, the impact may be more subtle or even go unnoticed. My husband for example, will admit that he may feel off or disconnected for days before he makes the connection between the symptoms in his body and whatever is happening in a relationship. Whether we experience it on a conscious level or not, the quality of our relationships have a direct and powerful impact on our physical and mental well-being.

Human Connection

Humans want to connect. It is our nature. According to Harville Hendrix, a nationally recognized couples therapist and bestselling author, "Connecting is our deepest desire, and to lose it is our deepest fear."[1] He is not just referring to the connection we feel with our partner alone but the connection we feel with any of our relations—child, sibling, co-worker, etc. Hendrix says that when we are not connected in our relationships, we experience anxiety. When we experience anxiety, we can be irritable, defensive, short-tempered, depressed, paranoid, etc. Everyone ends up suffering.

Not only do we want to be connected in relationships, there is evidence that we are connected to each other on levels much deeper than many of us have ever imagined. One of the biggest misconceptions we have about ourselves is that each of us is separate from one another, that we survive alone. Quantum physics tells us that we are far more interconnected at a subatomic level than we might imagine. This field demonstrates that there is no space between where one person ends and another begins. Our atoms are interchanging constantly. Our connection to each other is deep seeded, complicated, and very real. Our molecular connection has been shown to transmit energies like moods and attitudes between individuals.[2] A simple example of this happening is when we sense someone being sad, even if she isn't showing outward signs and we don't know the situation that is causing her sadness. We know she is sad because we sense it; we may even subtly or clearly feel it ourselves just by being in her presence. Recently I was with an old friend and I felt incredibly agitated, anxious, and unsettled in his presence. It was an unexpected feeling and perplexing to me. After learning more about this person's current life stressors and coping practices, it was clear that I was picking up on his agitated, anxious, and unsettled state. At Naropa, we called this phenomenon "exchange." We are literally exchanging mood, energies, and even thoughts with each other through our interconnected reality.

Experiencing positive connection with another person has a direct effect on the body and on health. It is a powerful healing agent for the body because it causes the release of a hormone called oxytocin—often referred to as the "love hormone" and most commonly known for its release during childbirth and breastfeeding. But the benefits of oxytocin are experienced much more often than just during birth and infancy. It is also released as a result of positive interactions and when receiving psychological support. High dose bursts occur with skin-to-skin contact, like hugs, snuggles, massages, love of a pet, and sex (orgasm in particular). Once present in the body, oxytocin decreases stress, anxiety, and depression. It decreases the level of the stress hormone cortisol and lowers our blood-pressure response to anxiety-producing events. As a result, the more oxytocin that our body releases the more able we are to deal with life stressors. Researchers have recently found that oxytocin infusion reduces cell death and inflammation in an injured heart and is thought to improve overall heart functioning. A study completed in Australia found that only 5 percent of people who went home to a dog after having a heart attack died within the year. However, 26 percent of people who returned to a home with no dog died within the year. The study contributed this survival difference to the benefits of oxytocin release from loving a pet.[3] Oxytocin has also been found to reduce cravings of drugs, alcohol, and sweets, increase sexual libido, enhance immune functioning, improve our ability to socialize and connect, promote sound sleep, and foster generosity. There is a cyclical effect with oxytocin: when we connect with others our body releases oxytocin, which then fosters more connection and generosity, which in turn keeps the oxytocin flowing, and the cycle advantageously continues. So, like with eating more kale, or stopping smoking, engaging in relationship in ways that facilitate oxytocin release can increase your health and the health of your family. Healthy relationships help us survive—literally. This understanding of how deeply the quality of our relationships can affect our health gives us more tools with which to build our "whole health" strategy.[4]

Loneliness

Perhaps to no one's surprise, relationship challenges impact us on emotional and social levels. What is striking is how these same struggles can affect us physiologically. Consider the opposite of connection—loneliness. When we are not connected, we may feel lonely or isolated. Recent research shows that beyond being an unpleasant experience, loneliness can actually harm the body's immune system by affecting a gene that controls immune functioning. Other scientists have discovered that lonely individuals produced more inflammation-related proteins in response to acute stress than did people who felt more socially connected. Many studies are now identifying a strong connection between loneliness and chronic stress, which as discussed, can lead to many health problems.[5]

To highlight the connection between loneliness and chronic stress I want to share a story about a group of individuals from Roseto, Pennsylvania. In the 1950s and 1960s, a group of Italian immigrants that lived in Roseto, Pennsylvania, were studied because they were noticed to have half the rate of heart disease than the rest of the country. At the time, scientists were eager to understand the causes of heart disease, and it was hoped that this group of individuals held the answers. Researchers naturally looked at diet first. These individuals ate meatballs fried in lard, pasta, and pizza. They drank a bottle of wine every night, and many smoked. The researchers quickly learned that their diet wasn't the answer to the heart disease question, so they moved on to genetics. They found that individuals that came from the same place in Italy, but lived in different parts of the United States, had the same rate of heart disease as the rest of the country—rejecting the DNA theory. The Roseto group was drinking similar water, had similar healthcare practices, and in general didn't have any health habits that set them apart from the rest of the country. The research team ended up concluding that the people of Roseto had half the rate of heart disease because no one in their community was ever lonely. They lived in multigenerational homes with kids, parents, and grandparents. They worked hard, but after work everyone would stop by each other's houses and visit. They would knock at each door, enter, and have a glass of wine. They gathered for multigenerational meals, went to the same church, and celebrated holidays together. If someone needed help, the community would jump in and offer assistance. I can picture their oxytocin continually flowing from all of this community-based connection. As the children from this community grew and went away to college, the community started disbanding. By the early 1970s, the people of Roseto had the same rate of heart disease as the rest of the country. What a great natural experiment this is to illustrate the power of healthy relationships. Conversely, when we don't prioritize relationships we can become lonely and overwhelmed, which results in physiological responses very similar to chronic stress.[6]

Interestingly, it may not be intuitive for many of us to even recognize loneliness when we experience it. We need to develop an understanding of loneliness in order to recognize it in ourselves. Recall how Hendrix claimed that when we are not connected we are anxious. Loneliness is merely the opposite of connection and when we are lonely we are anxious. When we lack regular companionship we don't feel seen, understood, or loved—we are lonely. Even the most introverted and independent of us need regular connection, whether it is from a pet, a partner, a family member, or even just one close friend. Just because we may be busy parents running all over town, interacting with people constantly, does not mean that we can't experience loneliness. In fact, our busyness can be the main contributing factor to our loneliness—and our anxiety. Loneliness is different than simply not being around people; rather, it is lacking connection with the people that we are with. Busyness and life stressors can distract us from true connection with the people around us. For me, becoming a new parent created many feelings of loneliness. When I had my oldest son, I often felt isolated, even though we lived in a big city. I was focused on my pursuit of figuring out parenting; I was exhausted from poor sleep; and my relationship with my husband was struggling as we tried to figure out our new life as parents together. From the outside, I'm sure coworkers and strangers couldn't tell I was lonely, but on the inside my tunnel vision as a new mom created barriers to my ability to connect with those close to me. During this time, I felt emotionally reactive in relationship with others and easily burdened by stressors. I did not feel well physically or emotionally and felt completely stuck in my inability to move through these challenges. Once I adjusted to motherhood, though, I found ways to connect meaningfully with people and my loneliness shifted so that I feel it less these days. I do still experience periods of loneliness, though. It usually comes on when I am overly busy with work, school, and family responsibilities. I am aware that when I am feeling isolated and lonely, I become more reactive in my home and stressors more easily bother me. I am now better able to recognize the feeling of loneliness and be proactive in reaching out to connect with my husband and others in my community when needed, nipping the unhealthy feeling in the bud. When thinking about the impact of loneliness on health, it is important to recognize that we get to choose the extent to which we engage in our community and nurture relationships. So as you tap into your individual experience with loneliness, note that small decisions we make on a daily basis can transform moments of loneliness or disconnect into moments of connection.

What We Focus on Grows

How can we use this knowledge about relationships and health to our advantage? First, you may have noticed in your life that the elements of your relationships that you focus on tend to grow or expand. If we focus on the ugly and annoying things that others do, we will get more ugliness magnified. For example, when I am in an irritable mood my husband's chewing of crunchy food can drive me crazy. After minutes (that seem like hours) of listening to the chewing, it is all I can hear. Nothing else in the world exists. The chewing gets louder, my nerves are on edge, and I feel my anxiety grow exponentially; I become annoyed at everything around me. I have a similar example with my dog. There are times when I have heightened awareness of all of the hair that he sheds in the house. When in this tunnel vision, all I see in the house and on my children's clothes is hair. I look at my dog, and all I can see is a nuisance. I cringe when people pet him as I imagine all the hair flying off his body. I become obsessed and edgy about other things that don't feel "in place" in my life. As easy as that, my relationship with my husband and my dog can contribute to persistent anxiety and stress. And we know what those can cause: inflammation and illness.

But, we have the power to make a healthier choice. Because when we focus on love, connection, and positivity, these grow. For example, when I notice and recognize how helpful it is when my husband cleans up after the dog or takes out the trash, my appreciation for him builds. As a result he is then often inspired to help around the house even more, and I am inspired to see all of the lovely things that he does well. With my children, if I praise the way they picked up toys or got dressed so quickly by themselves, I find my response encourages more of the same behaviors, and I actually notice more of their other positive behaviors as well. In contrast to the detrimental effects of focusing on irritations, focusing on positive elements of the relationship does not trigger an inflammatory response in the body. Rather it facilitates connection, release of oxytocin, and a general feeling of contentment and satisfaction.

Let's think about it from a neurochemical perspective. When I focus on the annoying chewing habits of my husband, my blood chemistry balance shifts from endorphins (peace hormones produced by the central nervous system and pituitary gland) to cortisol (stress hormone released in the adrenal cortex).[7] Typically, my comment to my husband about his chewing will evoke a defensive reaction from him, which then results in a change in his blood chemistry, reducing endorphins and increasing cortisol. The cycle rarely stops here. Recently, I raised my voice at my three boys when I walked into the playroom and found that they had oh so creatively mixed water and Play-Doh, making food in their play kitchen. The room was a sticky, slimy mess. I reactively yelled at them, expressing my frustration about the messy room. I'm sure I went on and on in an ugly voice. Later, while we all were cleaning up, my five-year-old said. "Mom, I don't like it when you yell at me. It doesn't feel good for my brain." From a neurochemical perspective, he was absolutely right. The chemicals that are released from fear and intimidation cause inflammation and emotional shutdown. Anxiety and fear don't feel good to the spirit and chemically add undue stress to the body.

Hendrix says it best: "What you do to another person you do to yourself."[8] He states that if you intimidate other people you create stress not only in them, but in yourself as well. If you bless another person, you create blessings in yourself as well. Being kind and generous to others supports our own health and well-being.

Family Dynamics

Let's look at how we can translate these concepts into tools that can improve the health of the family. Although the preceding concepts and the upcoming strategies apply to all of our relationships, the two primary relationships in the family system are the parent-child and the parent-parent relationships.

We all have moments when we express frustration, anger, irritation, and an endless list of other emotional reactions to our children in a less than skillful manner. It happens. We aren't perfect. However, the reality is that most of us in the United States jump into parenting without an inkling of prior experience, and most often without having even put much thought into parenting until the moment we are home with our newborn. We struggle to find the "right way" to parent, discipline, create structure, and end up with loving, caring, and respectful children. It can be a steep learning curve. This confusion often leads to yelling matches—like the Play-Doh mess—insensitive condemnations, or unreasonable demands. There is certainly no single answer for all of us (although everyone you ask, and every book you read, will have "an answer"). The reality for most of us is that without tools or methods for dealing with the endless challenging situations that come with parenting, we often fall back on instinctual behaviors in an attempt to maintain control and assert our authority. In some cases, we are lucky and those methods work. But more often they don't bring the result we want and don't nurture the type of relationship that we want with our children. As we begin to understand how the quality of our relationship affects our health, we see that the way we relate with our children has implications for our health and the health of our children. A fascinating study at Harvard University depicts the connection between physical health and the parent-child relationship. This study found that 98 percent of individuals who claimed that they were not loved by their parents had a major illness thirty-five years later. Only 24 percent of individuals who claimed that their parents did love them had a major illness in this same time frame.[9] These are sobering statistics that make us realize how important it is that our kids know—and believe—that they are loved by us. The credibility of our love is communicated largely by our actions and inevitably through our parenting style.

The intent of this section is not to convince you how to parent, but rather to help you discover the links between parenting, relating, and health, and to inspire you to explore and discover a set of tools and strategies that work for your parenting style. In my experience, the right tools can significantly reduce stress and improve relationships, with the nice side benefit of increasing oxytocin. There was a point when my husband and I felt like we were yelling at our kids too much and didn't have the "control" that we wanted. So we went to parenting classes offered by the local elementary school. The classes offered simple concrete tools that changed my parenting, and thus, my life. We learned techniques to show love and empathy to our children when they make mistakes instead of getting frustrated or yelling. We learned how to follow through with appropriate consequences so that they learn that personal decisions lead to natural consequences, both good and bad. It is important to remember that when we yell at our children their bodies react with "fight or flight" responses. Remember, these responses can cause cellular inflammation in the body when we experience it regularly. In addition, it can shut down the ability to learn and listen effectively. Therefore, children are less likely to "learn their lesson" when they are being yelled at or condemned. Thus, we perpetuate the cycle of the same frustrating behaviors. We need strategies to move from parenting that creates inflammation, to strategies that nurture love and relationship-building. If you often find yourself raising your voice or feeling out of control with your children, know that it is possible to do things another way. I know from experience. Improved parenting (relating) moves the whole family towards stronger "whole health."

The other primary relationship in the family system is that of parent to parent. It has its own unique challenges. Many relationships in modern society struggle with maintaining connection, especially as we become exhausted from the juggling act of everything we hold on our plate. Our ability to communicate openly and honestly may falter. Negativity can sneak its way into the relationship. Our deep seeded needs may start to express themselves in ways that are not healthy, affecting our personal health, as well as our family's health.

The ability of parents to relate and connect in a healthy manner is absolutely foundational to the health of the family. Everyone experiences significant stressors and health concerns if the people running the show are not cohesive and connecting in a healthy relationship. I know of a child who was in the middle of his parent's unfortunate conflict. When his dad drove away with the boy and his siblings to leave their mother, the five-year-old said, "I hope you and mom aren't going to ruin our lives forever." What a sad and sobering depiction of the deep impact parental discord has on children, and often for many years of their lives. As parents, it is easy to get so wrapped up in our relationship dramas and issues that we forget to take into account the impact of our reactions and interactions on our children. The role modeling that we provide regarding what healthy relationships look like should not be ignored or down-played. If we are struggling in our relationship with our partner, whether it is from subtle disconnect or outward conflict or rage, it is important to put attention into building effective communication skills in order to address these issues. Getting support from a counselor, taking time to get away together, or reaching out to a trusted community member for guidance are all ways that we can work on our adult relationships. Many parents realize that they are unable to connect in relationship with their partner anymore for a multitude of reasons. When we are faced with hard decisions about staying together or not, be aware that little ones are watching and learning about how to engage in difficult conversations. Even in these most extreme moments we have the opportunity to model respect and good communication. Professional counseling services can be a proactive way to enhance connection and good communication across the spectrum of disconnect--from resolving minor annoyances to managing heavy relationship issues.

Authenticity and Vulnerability

A common way in which disconnect can surface is through our resistance to being authentic. Deep down we all want to be fully seen for who we are, for our authentic selves. We desire this recognition from our partners, co-workers, parents, and friends. Yet we often fear that certain parts of our being are unlovable or unacceptable to others. We worry about being rejected—even by those who know us well, like our partners—if someone sees who we really are. This internal, often subconscious conflict can result in subtle, self-protective acts of inauthenticity—being fake, withdrawn, or passive aggressive. As we enact these defense mechanisms, we limit our ability to connect in our relationships.

I have become quite aware of my tendencies to be both authentic and inauthentic. I can be inauthentic when my ego needs people to see my professional capabilities, my clean home, my emotional intelligence, my "put-together" family, and my well-managed life. I hide by portraying an outward image of "having everything together." But living in this way is stressful, rigid, and smothering. One day I forgot to bring baked goods to a work party. I was talking to a colleague about this "atrocity," and I said, "I can't believe that I would forget something like that. Now people will see that I actually don't have it all together." The truth was, I didn't really feel bad about forgetting the treats. Rather, I felt humiliated that my co-workers might think that I can't juggle all of my responsibilities, that I might be perceived as unreliable. On the other hand, when I am in touch with my authentic self I find I am able to be vulnerable and show my husband, friends, co-workers, and neighbors that I can be scared, uncertain, fragile, and forgetful. When I'm connected authentically to myself, I feel comfortable with others knowing that I do not have my act together most of the time. When I am able to show up in that way, I feel much more confident, calm, and connected—to myself and to others. When we are able to be authentic, we act more naturally and it draws others in. My co-worker responded to my comment about the forgotten treats by saying, "Thank goodness other people do that too. I thought I was the only one that did that kind of stuff, and I have felt awful about myself when I forget things." Most often, our ability to be vulnerable and express ourselves authentically helps others also feel more comfortable shedding some of their own protective layers.

Allowing our true, authentic self to be fully seen by others requires a certain level of vulnerability. Best-selling author, social worker, and researcher Brene Brown has spent the last fifteen years studying vulnerability and authenticity. Vulnerability, she suggests, is having the courage to welcome uncertainty, risk, and emotional exposure.[10] Love, belonging, trust, joy, and creativity all require vulnerability. By tapping into this vulnerability, we are more able to authentically show up in relationships. The truth is, it takes a lot of mental energy to hide. When we show up we are more open to truly experience the most rewarding moments in life. The first step to being more authentic is to pay attention to the situations and relationships that typically cause us to stray from being who we truly are. Then, we should try to notice the moments and conditions that bring out our most authentic self. Brown so eloquently states:

> *Authenticity is a daily practice. Choosing authenticity means: cultivating the courage to be emotionally honest, to set boundaries, and to allow ourselves to be vulnerable; exercising the compassion that comes from knowing that we are all made of strength and struggle and connected to each other through a loving and resilient human spirit; nurturing the connection and sense of belonging that can only happen when we let go of what we are supposed to be and embrace who we are.*[11]

Practicing authenticity with our partner can be the safest place to begin. It may not always come naturally, but each time we open ourselves up we invite and welcome the same from our partner. This is the relationship that will reap the greatest rewards for our own health, as well as for the health of our whole family. Once vulnerability becomes more familiar in the family setting we are all then more able to take this practice into our other personal relationships.

Improving Communication

In addition to hiding our authentic self, we will also have moments of poor communication, mistrust, and arguments with people that we care about. It is an inevitable part of most relationships. The goal is not to completely avoid conflict or disagreements altogether, but rather to have awareness when disconnect occurs and strive to repair the relationship. In fact the ability to repair, which often requires some level of vulnerability, can actually lead to connection. Arguments are often about the same underlying issues: Did you hear me correctly?

Did you see me for who I am? And, did what I say mean anything to you? Hendrix offers four tips to help reduce the frequency and intensity of arguments and disconnect, and to increase our experiences of connection. These suggestions, along with other similar tools, can be used to improve communication and our ability to relate with our children, our significant other, and even other relationships that we have outside of the home.

Safe Conversation

One of the ways to support vulnerability and maintain connection with another is through enhancing one's sense of emotional safety. Without emotional safety, we feel anxious. When we are anxious we are defensive and protective, inhibiting our ability to be vulnerable and authentic. Thus, connection is interrupted. Remember, connecting is a key ingredient of our true nature, and we need it to optimize our health. However, to experience connection we require emotional safety. Hendrix teaches that emotional safety can be created through deep listening and deliberate conversation. Three specific tools can help us develop deliberate conversations that lead to safe and effective communication: mirroring, validation, and empathy.

> **Mirroring** is deep listening, where you tune into the other's internal story and turn off your own. After listening intently, you may respond "Let me see if I've got it. You said.... Did I get it? Do you want to share more?" When you mirror, you listen deeply to the other person's words and feelings and ask if you've understood correctly. The majority of the time we will be inaccurate when we attempt to reflect what one has just shared with us. When we are inaccurate it gives the other person the opportunity to clarify and help us understand correctly. It is challenging to listen to someone else's story, and especially the underlying feelings, because we naturally spend the majority of our time listening only to our own internal story line. To connect, we must let go of our own story so we can listen very carefully to the other's version of the story,

striving to see the way they see. Although this is a simple concept, it takes focus and intention to accomplish. A good general rule is to listen 80 percent of the time and talk 20 percent of the time.

Validation ultimately communicates, "I see your truth." You might respond by saying, "That makes sense to me," or "I can see how you see it that way." When we validate, we are acknowledging that the other's truth is as valid as ours. Validation is walking in another's shoes. You have to simply see the logic of others from their perspective. Every one of us thrives on validation.

Empathy means to relate to the feelings or experience that someone is having, "It sounds like you are feeling ___________." When we are listening to another's story, we should listen for both the content and any feelings that are being expressed. In other words, we should "read between the lines." We don't have to agree, and we can certainly have a different perspective, but we can show someone that we are able to see the world from his viewpoint and recognize his emotional experience. It is helpful to increase your emotional vocabulary so you can try to identify feelings accurately. Even if you guess the wrong feeling, the other person will have the opportunity to correct you and will likely feel grateful that you are trying to fully see and hear him.

Affirm and appreciate others

Appreciation means to increase another's value. When I share gratitude towards or compliment another person, I actually increase his or her value. As a result, they see themselves as valued, and I actually have heightened value for them. What a win-win! For example, I might say, "Honey, I just love the way you read books to our kids with so much animation." Or, "You are so amazing at helping with household chores without complaining." Or, "I just love the way you look in the clothes you are wearing today." The chemistry of our brains literally changes when we express appreciation to each other. In recognizing the power of expressing appreciation, my husband and I have committed to do this with each other regularly, and it has proven to be a powerful tool for staying connected and bringing us closer.

Be aware of what you look like when you listen

Pay attention to how you may look to the speaker the next time you are listening to someone. When we stare or glare at a speaker, our pupils get smaller and the amygdala—part of the limbic system of the brain that directs emotional reactions, memory, and decision making—of the person we are listening to subconsciously instructs her that we are not a person with whom he can feel safe and confident sharing openly. His body will automatically feel anxiety and go into defense mode to regulate and protect his vulnerability. Alternately, if we replace our glare with a relaxed gaze, the other person will feel like he can tell you anything. When we gaze our pupils are large and the recipient's amygdala reads this as "open" and "safe." A goal we can set for ourselves is to become a safe and welcome place for our spouse and children to share their vulnerable experiences, without anxiety or defenses.

Zero Negativity

Negativity is a destructive behavior that creates anxiety, which ends up blocking productive elements of relating, such as problem solving, romance, and general connecting. Unlike appreciation, negativity is how we devalue and put another person down. For example, I have repeatedly told my husband that he never cleans the food from the kitchen sink after doing the dishes. My tone is usually snappy and agitated. Negativity comes not necessarily from what we say but from how we say it. My request for the sink to be clean after washing dishes is not the issue; it is more that my tone implies that he or his behavior is inadequate. Practicing "zero negativity" means trying not to use any negativity in our interactions. Instead, we look at everything through the eyes of love. For example, I might focus on telling my husband what a great job he did doing the dishes and how lovely the kitchen looks, and that I appreciate his effort (using appreciation here to increase his value). I may or may not choose to add, "Would you mind cleaning the kitchen sink out when you get a chance? I'd appreciate it. Thanks again for doing the dishes." Sometimes I find that when I focus on appreciating him for doing the dishes I just end up cleaning out the sink myself, without resentment, because my heart is focused on gratitude.

Part of the goal of "zero negativity" is to live without judgment. When we are judging others, we are not nurturing love within ourselves or others. Judgment is the opposite of appreciation and love. It is devaluation. Love, on the other hand, is unconditional, positive appreciation. Love and judgment are incompatible modes of being. When we strive to remove negativity from every conversation, every interaction, with everybody at all times about everything, we begin to experience profound benefits of connection and health. Sounds impossible, right? Well, it might be. But, if we strive for no negativity we will at least slightly improve the love we share and decrease the judgment we have. We will also begin to increase our awareness of disconnected interactions with others and see opportunities to repair them. My husband and I practice catching disconnect caused by negativity by saying "ouch" to the person being negative. This gentle reminder gives us an immediate opportunity to redo the conversation with love and respect. Repairing interactions of disconnect is a primary tool for developing connection.[12]

☑ LIVE IT. MODEL IT. TEACH IT.

LIVE IT.

☐ We feel good when we are in harmony and connection with our partner and our children. We also reduce inflammation in our body and nurture health for ourselves and our families. Reflect on each of the relationships that you have in your home. Prioritize creating connecting interactions with all members of your family.

- [ ] Take time to reflect on your engagement with community. Are you satisfied with the level of support and connection that you have in your life? If not, brainstorm ways in which you can enhance your involvement with meaningful community.

- [ ] Notice how focusing your attention on connection and appreciation breeds more of the same, whereas focusing on negativity and disconnect produces more negativity and disconnect.

- [ ] Consider parenting classes to learn specific techniques for working with common challenges in raising children.

- [ ] Seek out professional marriage or family counseling for support and guidance if you want to make more dramatic improvements in your relationships—don't wait until small issues become major problems.

- [ ] Ask yourself about the level of authenticity and vulnerability present in your most meaningful relationships. Do you have room to improve how you truly show up in your relationships?

- [ ] Try Hendrix's four tips (safe conversation, affirm and appreciate others, be aware of what you look like when you listen, and zero negativity) to deepen your relationships and repair ruptured interactions when they arise in your home.

- [ ] Consider creating time in the week to have a family meeting where everyone in the family has a chance to voice his or her needs and wants. This consistent, weekly activity can help deepen relationships and tighten family cohesion. Have a fun activity or special treat during the meeting to increase the excitement of being together.

- [ ] Find time to connect with each family member one-on-one. Connecting happens on a deeper level when we can be fully present to an individual, which can be challenging to do in a group.

MODEL IT.

- [ ] Modeling what it looks and sounds like to connect in relationship is an invaluable life skill to pass on to your children. Children learn how to be in relationship by watching those closest to them. If we are stuck in a pattern of snapping at our partner, or using unloving words to communicate needs and wants, our children are learning that model. In turn, they will likely practice those same techniques habitually with the people that they love throughout their life. Conversely, they can learn that the depth of relationship and connection that we model with our spouse and with others close to us is the normal and appropriate way to interact. This is a big deal! Our modeling sets them up for success or failure on the relationship front, and chronic health or chronic inflammation on the physical front.

- [ ] When you feel lonely, model to your children what it looks like to reach out to others in order to build companionship and connection.

- [ ] Model vulnerability and authenticity by fully showing up in your relationships as your true self. When being vulnerable, consider sharing with your children in the moment what it feels like to be vulnerable. Demonstrate the courage it takes to show up in this way and allow them to witness the many benefits.

- [ ] Show them what it looks like and feels like to have effective conversations, to be appreciated and valued, to be received lovingly, and to not be judged through verbal and nonverbal forms of communication. Talking negatively about other people may teach them that it is okay to talk about others negatively and will suggest to them that you likely have negative and judgmental thoughts about them as well.

TEACH IT.

- [ ] Teach your children about oxytocin and how powerful it is in the body. At our house, when we give our kids hugs or snuggles we will often make an exciting ordeal about the oxytocin that we feel pumping in our bodies. Sometimes we fall over backwards to show how much oxytocin we feel. My five-year-old son has oxytocin in his vocabulary; I grin inside when I hear him use it.

- [ ] Help your children recognize the experience of loneliness and help them discover ways to foster connection during those times.

- [ ] Talk to your children about the benefits of authenticity and vulnerability in relationships. Acknowledge the courage required to be their true selves.

- [ ] Teach your family the components for safe conversation: mirroring, validation, and empathy.

- [ ] Teach your children feeling words at a very young age so they have the ability to express their own emotions effectively, to listen for emotions in others, and be able to validate others' feelings. We try to name our emotions and help our children do the same. For example, when one of the boys is whining a lot, I might say, "I'm feeling frustrated listening to all of the fussing this morning. It is draining my energy." This helps them understand my emotions and build their feeling vocabulary.

- [ ] Explain to your older children how their body language and subtle shifts in eye expression affects the listening experience of others.

- [ ] Point out examples in life where others have been devalued or valued by the words and actions of another. Demonstrate how to value others.

- [ ] Teach your family what fundamental connection is and that above all we want to strive to love, share, encourage, and appreciate each other. Help them understand that negativity is toxic and that being mean to others has health consequences for them.

6

Regular Physical Activity and Adequate Sleep

Exercise and maintaining proper sleep are cornerstones of good health. Ignoring the importance of exercise and proper sleep can have a dramatically negative impact on your longevity and other health indicators, to the point even of negating the efforts you put into your diet. This chapter will focus on why we need to keep our body moving and allow our body stillness.

Move Your Body

Most of us know that exercise improves heart and lung functioning, helps with weight loss, and strengthens muscles. We may or may not appreciate that it also reduces our risk of major diseases, stimulates the growth of new brain cells, improves digestion, and adds years to our lives. The physiological and psychological benefits of physical activity are vast and not yet all completely understood.

You have probably heard advice that you should exercise thirty minutes a day, or sixty minutes every other day, or seven minutes per day, or some other ideal amount of time in order to be healthy. You can find any number of sources to give expert advice on the amount of time you should spend exercising. My goal is not to tell you what you need to do but rather to inspire you to appreciate the multitude of benefits achieved from exercise and movement.

There are significant psychological benefits to physical activity. Exercise releases chemicals in the body called endorphins. These endorphins interact with the receptors in your brain that reduce your perception of pain.[1] Endorphins also trigger a positive feeling in the body, similar to the effect of morphine. Runners often refer to this feeling as "runner's high," but any form of exercise can help give our mood a boost when we are feeling down or overwhelmed. Exercise improves self-esteem and even reduces symptoms of depression or anxiety. Individuals who exercise also tend to feel better about their bodies even if they see no physical changes.

Most of us don't realize the extent to which exercise is important to our physical well-being. In addition to improving heart and lung health, developing muscle strength, and losing weight, routine physical activity can also:

Balance hormones: Exercise reduces insulin levels and increases serotonin. Moderating insulin is important in controlling inflammation and overall health, and regulating serotonin levels can help boost a low mood as well as relieve depression as effectively as antidepressant medication in many individuals.

Strengthen the immune system: People who exercise have a healthier balance of bacteria in their gut (see Chapter 11 for details on the importance of gastrointestinal microflora). In addition, moderate workouts temporarily rev up the immune system by increasing the activity of our "fighter" immune cells.

Increase longevity: Studies have shown that being active cuts the risk of premature death nearly in half for both men and women.

Prevent heart problems: You may have heard, exercise is the best way to increase HDL. HDL is a component of cholesterol that is protective to our cardiovascular system and high levels are a significant contributor to heart health. Physical activity can also reduce arterial inflammation, a risk factor for heart attacks and stroke.

Control blood sugars: Exercising uses up sugar circulating in the body and lowers hormones (like insulin) that store those sugars as fat and cause inflammation.

Protect against cancer: Exercise may reduce the risk of colon cancer by speeding the movement of waste through the gut and lowering insulin levels. It may also protect against breast and prostate cancer by regulating hormone levels.

Combat stress: Physical activity lowers levels of stress hormones. It increases energy and improves mood, releases feel-good endorphins, and acts as a meditative-like practice that helps focus our attention on one task. Stress damages the hippocampus, an area of the brain responsible for memory and many other essential functions. Raising our heart rate through exercise can reverse the damage to the brain that is caused by stress.

Improve neurologic function: Exercise has been shown to help improve memory, learning, and cognitive functioning. Some studies have even shown that exercise may make us smarter.

Improves circulation: Exercise improves blood circulation to muscles and promotes a more efficient way to deliver nutrients to the body. Exercise helps move the nutrients you receive from your healthy eating habits to the parts of the body where they are needed.[2]

I am the first to admit that incorporating regular exercise into my daily life is the hardest of the health components for me. There have been only a few periods in my life when I was exercising consistently. I have never really enjoyed exercising, and I am easily discouraged by the fatigue, discomfort, and exertion that can accompany it. It is easy for me to blame lack of time, the cost of classes, and my husband's inconsistent work schedule for not being able to exercise. Finding the right form of exercise that suits me is an ongoing challenge. If you are already inclined towards exercise you can breeze through the next section. But if you struggle with exercise like I do, you may need to be a little creative in thinking about how to get your body moving.

We are all familiar with the most common forms of exercise like running, biking, spinning and Zumba classes, swimming, tennis, yoga, etc., but remember that you don't have to run ultra-marathons to get your heart rate up. Some examples of moderate exercise that may be good solutions for the exercise-averse include:

- Dancing (with your kids)
- Rollerblading (with your kids)
- Hiking (with your kids)
- Jumping on a trampoline (with your kids)
- Wrestling with your kids (or your partner...wink, wink!)
- Gardening
- Golf (without a cart)
- Housework, especially mopping, sweeping, running up and down the stairs cleaning, or vacuuming
- Brisk walking to the grocery store, in the mall, or around the block during lunch breaks
- Taking the stairs at every opportunity
- Yard work, especially mowing, raking, or shoveling snow
- Having fun tracking your steps with a pedometer

As with many lifestyle changes we often need to start with baby steps. The good news is that there is some fascinating research coming out that suggests that simply incorporating more non-exercise movement into our day can have significant health benefits, potentially more benefits than active exercise. So for parents like me who resist regular exercise the starting point doesn't have to be running five miles a day. Taking a look at our daily activities and the amount of time we are sedentary is a good starting point. Although aerobic exercise is proven to have positive health benefits across the board, new research highlights the health benefits of simply moving more throughout the day. This is due to the fact that we, as a society, have become significantly more sedentary in the last few decades as technology has made many jobs more efficient and computer based. Many of us may easily spend over thirteen hours of our day in a sedentary position.[3] Increased sedentary work and lifestyle activities have been associated with multiple health problems, including weakened bones, ligaments, and muscles, core muscle imbalance, joint deterioration, weight gain, deep vein thrombosis, reduced sperm count, and cardiovascular disease.[4] Prolonged sitting appears to have negative effects on fat and cholesterol metabolism and be correlated to mortality. One of the most striking findings about these implications of a sitting lifestyle is that they are found to affect all sedentary people similarly, even when individuals meet current recommended exercise levels. Translation: running every day after work does not make up for sitting in a chair for eight hours a day.[5]

Therefore, simply focusing on reducing overall sedentary time, as well as breaking up sedentary tasks, can have significant health implications. This is especially pertinent for those who work in an office environment that may require computer work for the majority of the day. For those of us parents who spend a lot of the day managing children, being sedentary may not be the problem. With three children, five years old and under, I find that I am rarely sitting still. Between cleaning the house, doing laundry, managing yard work, running up and down the stairs to wipe tears or break up a fight, I am moving constantly. Yet as technology becomes more integrated into our lives and many influences in modern life draw us towards a more sedentary lifestyle, it is important even for active parents to be aware of the negative health implications of a sedentary lifestyle. Here are some simple strategies to increase your non-exercise activity levels:

1. If you work at a computer, get up and walk away from your workstation (to the bathroom or to get a drink) at least once an hour. Walk briskly and swing your arms to activate more muscles and burn more calories. You might have to set a timer as a reminder at the beginning.
2. Stand at your work station for a few minutes or more every half hour. Stand while talking on the phone. Pace, sway, bend, stretch, swing. Look into purchasing or building a standing desk.

3. Carve out time for more walking. During work breaks walk as far as you can and get outside if possible.
4. Climb stairs instead of taking the elevator.
5. Park your car at the far end of the parking lot instead of seeking the closest parking place.
6. Increase outdoor meeting and working spaces.
7. Set up more active meeting room environments—like standing height conference room tables or interactive-based meetings, for example.

Although there is evidence that the non-exercise physical activity I get as a parent is beneficial, I am not going to give up my pursuit of regular aerobic exercise. The physical and mental health benefits of aerobic activity are clear. But starting by simply increasing movement during daily life moves me in the right direction.

If you have not exercised in a while check with your doctor, health coach, or a personal trainer and start slowly. If you are motivated to exercise by a desire to lose weight, please realize that you are unlikely to lose weight unless you also change what you are eating. Exercise for the benefit of exercise, not only to lose weight, or you may be setting yourself up for disappointment. In time, you will increase your muscle mass, decrease your body fat, change your shape, balance hormones, and more importantly, lower your insulin levels, your average blood sugar levels, your inflammatory markers, and, therefore, lower your risk of most diseases of the modern world.

Rest Your Body

Resting your body is just as important as moving it. People in the United States are getting less sleep than ever before. According to the National Sleep Foundation, middle-aged Americans sleep on average one hour less than we did fifty years ago, and the number of people sleeping less than six hours per night is increasing.[6] On average, we get about six and a half hours of sleep per weeknight.[7] According to the National Geographic documentary *Sleepless in America*, we are not getting enough sleep and our chronic sleep deprivation causes irreversible damage to our health. Forty percent of Americans are sleep deprived, many getting less than five hours of sleep per night. These trends are likely due to environmental factors, such as the need to work more, rather than to any biological change in our need for sleep. Most of us do not fully appreciate all the ways in which sleep deprivation affects our health, and therefore easily disregard its importance in the face of other demands: long work days, multiple jobs, needs of children, household tasks, etc. Interestingly, adolescents are among the most sleep deprived. This is a problem for our children whose health is critical while they are active, learning most of the day, and need to be creative and innovative as they navigate their world. High school students who sleep more have higher test scores and lower rates of depression.[8] No matter the age, most of us devalue rest so much that we feel we can "steal" from our sleep time when we are overwhelmed by other demands and priorities.

When we experience sleepiness we usually know we are over-tired, but most of us do not understand the connections that sleepiness has to many negative health concerns. We simply fuel up with coffee or energy drinks and push through. Many people even pride themselves on how little sleep they need to function. But poor sleep is nothing to be proud of. Poor sleep quality and short sleep duration are associated with higher levels of inflammation and illness. Sleep should truly be one of the cornerstones of our health strategy for the family. Medical science confirms that sleep is critical for stress, weight management, and overall health.

The average amount of sleep that you need to maintain alertness on a daily basis is called your "sleep need" and is typically seven to nine hours per night. When you get less than your sleep need you build up what is called "sleep debt." If you build up more than twenty hours of sleep debt you may not be able to reverse the long-term effects of sleep deprivation.[9] Thus, you can easily imagine how chronic sleep problems can lead to long-term health problems.

After a poor night of sleep, most of us have had the experience of finding ourselves less patient with a child or spouse, more sensitive to things not going our way, etc. Sleep helps our body recover from the day and repair itself through cell, muscle, and tissue growth. Research shows that sleep greatly affects our mood, irritability, anxiety, concentration, memory, and ability to interact socially. And, of course, our mood affects how we function throughout the day. When we have an appropriate amount of rest, we tend to be happier, have fewer negative reactions, and are able to access pleasant memories more easily.[10] Perhaps most importantly, our happier, rested selves are much more effective at implementing and maintaining the practices that allow for whole health.

In addition to affecting our mood, sleep deprivation prematurely ages us by interfering with the production of growth hormones, which are released by our pituitary glands during deep sleep (as well as during certain types of exercise).[11] Growth hormones help us look and feel younger. If you want to get rid of those circles under your eyes or slow the development of wrinkles—sleep can do it!

Although wrinkles and a little moodiness may seem like a tolerable price to pay in the scope of life's demands and challenges, the effects of sleep deprivation can actually be more severe. Interrupted or impaired sleep has been associated with increases in illness and inflammation. Short duration sleepers (especially those getting less than six hours of shuteye a night) are at higher risk for infection, insulin resistance, obesity, diabetes, cardiovascular disease, cancer, arthritis, depression, and mood disorders. Research has shown poor sleep to have the following adverse effects on health:[12]

> *Weakened immune system:* Poor sleep can make us more prone to catching colds and flus because it decreases T lymphocytes and increases inflammatory markers, suppressing immune system functioning. In one study, people who slept less than six hours per night had 50 percent less resistance to viral infection than those getting eight hours of sleep.[13] In another study, young adults who had been given a flu shot after four nights of reduced sleep had less than half of the antibody response ten days later, compared with individuals having normal sleep at the time of vaccination. Conversely, adequate sleep can help keep our immune systems primed for attack.[14]

Heightened emotions: The amygdala of the brain controls basic emotions like fear and anger. The frontal cortex plays a key role in emotions. Sleep is vital for the function of the frontal cortex. When rested, your frontal cortex communicates nicely with your amygdala and essentially acts as a break to your emotional gas pedal. When we are sleep deprived there is disconnect between these two brain centers, allowing emotions to take over.

Slowed reaction time: When we're not well rested, we do not react as quickly as we normally would, making driving or other safety related activities dangerous. One study found that driving while tired was just as dangerous as drinking and driving.[15]

Accelerated tumor growth: Quality of sleep is as important as the amount. Research shows poor quality sleep, including frequent waking, can speed cancer growth, increase the disease's aggressiveness, and dampen the immune system's ability to control early cancers. Tumors grow two to three times faster in laboratory animals with severe sleep dysfunctions, primarily due to the lack of melatonin production which would otherwise discourage cancer growth.[16]

Pre-diabetic state: A full night's sleep may help prevent diabetes. A study at the University of Chicago involving healthy young men with no risk factors for diabetes found that after just one week of inadequate sleep, they were in a pre-diabetic state.[17]

Heart disease: Poor sleep habits have been linked to heart disease. One thread connecting sleep and heart disease is inflammation. Poor sleep increases C-reaction protein (causing inflammation), as well as activates the sympathetic nervous system's "fight or flight" response (causing more stress hormones).[18]

Cancer: Insulin resistance, shifted cortisol levels, and disrupted melatonin production caused by poor sleep are three significant factors that increase the risk of cancer. One study showed that women who exercised regularly and were generally healthy had a 47 percent higher risk of cancer if they were sleeping fewer than seven hours a night. Researchers at Stanford University also found that good sleep habits can be a valuable weapon in fighting cancers, citing melatonin and cortisol production as vital players in patient recovery. One study found that men who had trouble sleeping were twice as likely to develop prostate cancer as those who slept well. Other studies have suggested night shift workers to have higher rates of cancer. They are also more likely to have "shifted cortisol rhythms," in which their cortisol levels peak in the afternoon rather than the morning.[19]

Impaired cognition: Sleeping less than six hours a night can impact your ability to think clearly the next day. In one study, mice that were deprived of sleep lost 25 percent of the neurons located in the brain associated with cognitive processes. Sleep deprivation reduces our ability to process information and make decisions.[20]

Impaired memory: Studies continue to show how important quality sleep plays in learning and memory. Sleep affects learning in two ways. First, lack of sleep impairs a person's ability to focus and learn efficiently. Secondly, sleep is necessary to make a memory "stick" so that it can be recalled later. Even a single night of poor sleep—four to six hours—can impact your ability to think clearly the next day and impair your performance on physical or mental tasks.[21]

Sleep and nutrition are intricately related. Researchers have found that people who sleep five hours per night have a 50 percent higher chance of being obese, while those who sleep six hours have a 23 percent greater risk than those who receive adequate sleep. Less sleep is associated with an almost two-fold increase in obesity, a trend that can be detectable in children as young as five.[22] Animals faced with food shortage or starvation sleep less; conversely, animals subjected to total sleep deprivation for prolonged periods of time increase their food intake markedly.[23] Poor sleep contributes to day time fatigue which can lead to reduced activity and weight gain. Poor sleep reduces the fat regulating hormone leptin and increases levels of the hunger hormone ghrelin. The resulting increase in hunger and appetite can easily lead to overeating and weight gain. In addition, when we are not sleeping we have more opportunity to eat and often choose high caloric food out of boredom or stress. All of these factors contribute to weight gain and eventually obesity.

In addition to the association of short sleep durations and numerous health problems, most concerning is the strong link between sleep deprivation and an increased risk of death. Epidemiological and lab studies suggest that short sleep is associated with increased risk of metabolic disorders, which likely contributes to the increased mortality rates associated with short sleep duration. Research has shown that those who get seven to eight hours of sleep have lower mortality rates than those who sleep fewer hours (less than seven hours).[24]

Now you've heard the bad news about sleep deprivation and sleep debt. As with any challenge, the key to getting better sleep is recognizing the factors that influence the quality and amount of sleep we get. This understanding allows us to take small steps towards improved sleep habits and the associated health benefits. In addition, appreciating that getting more sleep will ultimately help us be more productive and effective during our waking hours can help motivate us to make the changes needed. The good news is that there are many natural techniques that can help you restore sound sleeping habits. And there is evidence that people who originally slept less than seven to eight hours each night, but then changed behaviors and increased sleep, also have lower mortality rates than those who continue to sleep fewer hours.[25]

The following are a few simple, practical methods that can have a significant impact on your sleep.

Sleep in a dark room: Even the tiniest bit of light in the room can disrupt your pineal gland's production of melatonin. Melatonin is responsible for creating your circadian rhythm, or biological clock. Cover your windows and turn off night lights if you are able. If you need a light, install a low-wattage yellow, orange, or red light bulb.

Get some sun: Your circadian rhythm needs light. Ten to fifteen minutes of sunlight will let your internal clock know that daylight has arrived, making it less confused by weaker light signals during the night. Do your best to get outdoors daily for thirty to sixty minutes during the brightest portion of the day.

Take a hot bath one and a half to two hours before bedtime: This increases your core temperature and when you get out of the bath tub the resulting rapid drop in body temperature can signal to your body that you are ready for sleep.

Know your biological sleep clock: Most people's melatonin release peaks around nine or ten at night. Falling asleep is easiest during peak melatonin releases. When your melatonin peaks you will likely feel a rush of fatigue and start feeling ready for bed. If we go to bed after our melatonin peaks it is harder for us to fall asleep and get into deep levels of sleep. Pay attention to your own biological sleep clock, which is probably in tune with going to bed around nine or ten. Try to go to bed and wake up at the same time every day.

Keep the temperature in your bedroom below seventy degrees Fahrenheit: Studies show that the optimal room temperature for sleep is quite cool, between sixty and sixty eight degrees. Keeping your room cooler or hotter can lead to restless sleep.

Avoid watching TV or using your computer, or other light-emitting electronic gadgets, at least two hours before going to bed: The light in these devices tricks your brain into thinking it is still daylight, affecting melatonin production, which has a direct correlation with our ability to fall asleep. This explains why I have a hard time falling asleep on nights when I work late on the computer.[26]

Identify physiological barriers that negatively impact sleep: Some common physiological factors that affect sleep are hormone imbalances—especially in perimenopausal and menopausal women—thyroid problems, uncontrolled stress and anxiety, poor diet, food sensitivities, and imbalances in the intestinal flora, to name a few. It is a good idea to seek the help of a trusted naturopath or medical doctor versed in non-pharmaceutical sleep interventions to identify and address the root cause.

Get your kids to STOP waking you up at night: Up to half of all toddlers and one third of all preschoolers in the U.S. still wake at least once at night. Therefore, it is safe to assume that I am not the only one whose sleep is affected by children.[27]

This last point is worth delving into further because it is a significant barrier to sleep for many families. Before I had kids I thought it was ridiculous when I heard stories about children not sleeping through the night. I figured that parents were doing something to create such obnoxious patterns, and it was their own fault for creating monsters. My mother always told me that my siblings and I slept through the night after nine months, and that sleep was never an issue in our house. Well, much to my surprise, great sleeping kids have not been my experience. Even though I tried tirelessly to avoid "negative sleep habits" when my kids were infants, sleep has turned out to be one of my biggest challenges as a parent. If we have a night during which no child wakes at some point, we celebrate in the morning as if we won the lottery. Most nights consist of our youngest waking up to potty at least once, feeling scared once or twice, and needing to be tucked in at least once. These events are combined with the random pee accident or nightmare that causes a frantic ordeal from one of the older boys. I do not sleep six to eight consecutive hours most nights, and I haven't for over five years. This reality of parenting young children in today's society has been a major concern for our family's health and well-being.

Research shows how important it is to get six to eight hours of sleep at night, with each individual having his own required amount. My personal observations confirm that when I sleep six to eight consecutive hours at night I feel more energetic and alert, and think more clearly. However, my cumulative sleep debt can make me feel like I walk around half-dead most of the time. Every step we can take towards improving our children's sleep habits will go miles towards improving our sleep and the overall health of the whole family.

It is not only beneficial for us parents to have sleeping children, but it is critical for our children to get adequate sleep—from preschool through college. In order to thrive, children need to have energy to focus, concentrate, retain information, be creative problem-solvers, and control impulses. Sleep is essential for these skills.[28] The National Sleep Foundation recommends the following steps to help increase your children's sleep:

> *Turn off electronics while children sleep:* On average, children with electronics on in their bedroom get about an hour less of sleep compared to those who don't. Light from electronic devices interferes with sleep. Their room should be completely dark as their pineal glands are affected by night lights.
>
> *Be a good role model:* Parents with electronic devices in their own bedroom are more likely to have kids who have them.
>
> *Enforce bedtime rules:* Children with a set bedtime and set rules about how late they can watch TV, use cell phones, or drink caffeinated drinks, sleep an average of up to an hour more than children whose parents do not have rules. Consistency is critical.

Reduce evening activities and homework: Performing better in fewer activities can be a healthy trade for trying to do too many activities while fatigued. Try not to let homework interfere with your established bedtime rules.[29]

Here are some strategies that have worked for my husband and me as we strive for better sleep:

Sleeping in the guest bedroom: When we have a particularly challenging trend of sleep debt accumulation, we take turns getting a good night sleep in the guest bedroom. When I'm in the guest bedroom, I turn on the fan, put earplugs in, and check out until morning. Because my husband travels so regularly, he is able to get consecutive sleep during his work trips (most of the time). When he comes home, he helps with night duty so I can get some sleep.

Sleeping space in our room: We have made our bed a place where parents sleep—not kids—because that is what works best for our sleeping needs. We have created a couple of beds on the floor of our room and our rule is that kids who come into our room quietly and do not wake up the parents can sleep in the bed on the floor. If kids wake up the parents, they go back to their room to sleep. Sometimes we wake and there are kids on the floor, and we don't know when or how they came in because they were so quiet.

Early bedtime: I am often conflicted at eight or nine o'clock at night when I am exhausted and ready for bed yet craving time to myself without little people pulling on me, whining at me, or just needing this or that from me. I love my evening time. But I try to hit the hay by ten, even if I am jazzed about a project, movie, or downtime. I wish I could get myself to bed earlier on a regular basis, but as I balance the need for personal time, a ten o'clock bedtime has become a good compromise.

Tokens: I always ask parents how they deal with sleep issues in their home. It is validating to hear that the sleep issues that many parents have parallel mine, and it is informative to hear about what parents are trying and what is working to increase their children's sleep. One mother shared with me the success she has had with using tokens to get her children to sleep, so we integrated that strategy at our house. When my children sleep through the night without waking parents, they receive a token (they also receive tokens for other things like getting up and dressing themselves without being asked). They can turn their tokens in for various prizes; for example, three tokens equals a snack when it is not snack time, five tokens equals one-on-one time with mom or dad, ten tokens equals fifteen minutes of a game on the iPad, etc. It seems that tokens cured my middle child's obsession with waking during the night, as he rarely wakes us at night now that we have implemented the token reward system in our house.

Talk to kids about the rules and options for sleep: It can be helpful to talk to your children about the importance of sleep and the needs of parents to sleep well too. Some kids will sleep better at night after merely explaining to them the benefits for the kids and the parents. Don't underestimate your small child's ability to understand daily practices and habits. After having a horrific trend of screaming night wakings from my middle child, one night I told him, "I hope you have a good night tonight, feel free to scream and cry in the middle of the night if you need to." He looked at me puzzled and he said, "If I scream and cry I would wake up my brothers." I said, "Oh, I won't let that happen. I will come and shut your door, so they can't hear. If you need something from me, feel free to come into my room quietly and ask for help." That night he came into our room quietly and whispered to us that he needed to go to the bathroom. It was a miracle!

Sleep training clock: We use a clock that tells the kids when they can get out of bed in the morning. It is set for seven, and they know that they can only get out of bed in the morning when the clock is yellow. It works like magic for those early wakers! If one of the kids wakes before the training clock indicates that it is time, we simply put him back in his room and tell him he can get out of bed when it is time.

Exercise and Sleep

Increasing exercise and getting more sleep can sound like overwhelming objectives for most of us. Both require more time, right? There is some good news on this front. Evidence suggests that exercise helps improve sleep. The more we exercise, the better we sleep. Adequate rest then enhances the energy and motivation that we need to move our bodies and be active. Sleep and exercise end up being a perfect feedback loop.

☑ LIVE IT. MODEL IT. TEACH IT.

LIVE IT.

- ☐ Reflect on your exercise and sleep patterns. In what ways can you improve? Experiment with how to make exercise and good sleep a priority in your life.

- ☐ Try to come up with a regular routine for physical activity that includes an activity that you enjoy. If you are like me and have a hard time finding exercise that you love, then find a way to move your body regularly and start out slow so you set yourself up for long-term follow through and success.

- ☐ Remember how important sleep is for your health, and strive to meet your sleep need each night.

MODEL IT.

- ☐ Show your family the importance of exercise by being physically active in front of them. If you always exercise before they wake up or while they are at school, they may not know that you value it. If you exercise when they are not around, talk about your exercise regimen openly with them.

- ☐ Exercise together. One thing that has encouraged me to get on our elliptical is making an activity out of it with my kids. I have put on an exercise show for them, and I exercise on the elliptical right next to them. We also play exercise-based board games and share in fun and laughter while moving our bodies.

- ☐ Going to bed at an appropriate time and demonstrating to your kids the importance of sleep will help them see the value that you put on sleep and influence how they view the importance of sleep in their lives.

TEACH IT.

- ☐ Talk to your kids about the importance of exercise and sleep. Teach them the benefits of an active life with adequate rest as well as the disadvantages of ignoring these healthy lifestyle habits.

7

Connecting to Your Spirit

A solid grounding in who we are and connecting to our spirit is the final primary food in the pursuit of whole health. Connecting to our spirit fuels what we do and how we live—and has a direct impact on how we take care of ourselves, how we view our work, how we eat, how we exercise, and how we relate to others. We are best able to serve the world when we truly know ourselves. Knowing our deeper self elevates our awareness that we are called to be more than just an employee or a parent. In Chapter 4, we considered the importance of living an undivided life and finding value in the work that we do. Increasing our self-awareness makes it more and more difficult to continue living a divided life. We come to know our true self, which in turn naturally directs us to our calling and purpose. This is what connecting to your spirit is all about. It is tuning in to our inner voice which guides us to the best decisions for ourselves, our families, and our communities. But we must learn to listen to that inner voice first. When we ignore it, we more easily experience challenges, make mistakes, and develop unhappy patterns. In fact, living in a way in which we listen to and honor our inner self is the key to true happiness. Our connection with ourself and with that which is bigger than us is much more important than what we do for a living. But building this awareness of purpose and finding a connection to our true self is not easy. The purpose of this chapter is to reinforce the value of our spiritual connection and to offer suggestions to help you get closer to knowing your true self. Clearly we all have our own spiritual paths. Your path can play a key role in helping you discover your purpose in life and ultimately become a powerful link to bring "whole health" to you and your family.

Unfortunately, for many busy parents with full plates, the primary food that gets the shortest shrift is connecting to spirit. We may blame lack of time, but I believe the barriers run deeper and include our underlying fear of knowing ourselves and of being vulnerable, and the unnatural feeling of slowing down when we are used to moving and doing.

What is Our Spirit?

I think of spirit as our innermost self, our truest essence, the part of us present when we close our eyes, escape our thoughts and just rest in that intangible being that lives within us. It is the part of us with no judgment, ego, competition, fear, or doubt. When we can connect to this part of our being, we begin to have clarity about what is right for us and to feel in tune with our values. We trust the direction our lives are taking. When we trust the deeper purpose in our lives, even mortality becomes less scary. Truly coming to know ourselves can be an elusive challenge. Specific practices and tools can help guide us down a path that leads to connection with our true selves.

There are endless ways to connect with our spirit. Many people connect with their spirit through religion. They go to church, mass, or temple, become inspired, and feel completely in touch with their inner most self. Although church may be a place where many people connect to their spirit, connection to spirit often occurs through other experiences and places too. Some people connect with their spirit by being in nature, doing art, playing music, or meditating. How we understand our connection to our spirit is for each of us to discover. How, where, or with whom is not what matters. Finding our own way and becoming inspired by the insights that our true self reveals is the spiritual journey. When we recognize that connecting to our spirit influences our deeper connection to life we see that spirit and health are inseparable.

What connects you to your spirit? What do you do to take care of yourself and to know yourself deeply? What experiences leave you feeling high and unconcerned about the minor details in life? When do you feel like you are part of something, connected to purpose and community? For me funerals and weddings bring out this sense of connection to deeper purpose. The big things that matter become very clear, and the minor struggles and challenges fall off my radar. Connecting with close friends in meaningful conversations and reflecting on life and death also help me connect to my true self. Paying attention to what elicits these experiences and moments in our life can guide us to the tools we need to maintain connection on a regular basis. There are countless tools that can guide us to regular connection with our spirit. Here are some that have worked for me—and for many others.

Slowing Down

In most cases, slowing down is fundamental to facilitating a strong connection to our spirit. Everyone slows down and connects in different ways. Buddhists practice sitting meditation. Christians practice prayer. But while many of our spiritual communities offer practices that help us become more centered and tuned in to our inner spirit, it can be hard for many of us to actually integrate these "slowing" practices into our daily life. We are simply so busy that being still can actually feel awkward and scary. Who can blame us? Our "to-do" lists are never ending. This busyness reinforces the misconception that if we aren't doing, moving, or completing tasks, then we are wasting time. Paradoxically, though, when we carve out time to slow down and find the things that connect us to our truest expression, we in turn put more focused and efficient effort into the things that actually matter to us. We waste less time doing mindless, petty, or meaningless tasks. Taking the time for slowness can actually make us more productive!

A close friend started a new family ritual called, "Sabbatical Sunday." I love this concept! On Sabbatical Sunday, everyone in the family "unplugs" from the phone, Internet, and television, and they spend the day playing games with each other, reading, hanging out, and engaging in things that help them slow down, be less distracted, and actually be in relationship with each other and their inner selves. I am excited to start this ritual in our house to create a structured way for our family to slow down and pay attention to what really matters on a regular basis.

My husband enthusiastically shares how his experiences bow hunting connects him so closely to nature and himself. He talks about the silence, the beauty, hearing his own breath, being in touch with all the life that surrounds him, walking so slowly and with such purpose, and being completely tuned in to every sound, smell, noise, and sight around him. No other experience brings him closer to feeling truly alive and connected than those moments. It is his way of slowing down, connecting to self, and coming out refreshed and more in tune with his deeper values. As hard as it is for me when he leaves for long stretches to go hunting, I hear the importance of this deep connection he has, and I support and encourage these experiences. We all need to find our way of "investing" in slowness and connection in order to bring their benefits to the rest of our lives.

Mindfulness Practices

Mindfulness practices help us focus attention on our emotions, thoughts, and sensations occurring in the present moment. Meditation is one type of mindfulness practice. Others are yoga, tai chi, qigong, centering prayer, and chanting. Even though meditation has its roots in Buddhism, secular practices of focusing on attention have been found to be beneficial for physical and mental wellness. Mindfulness meditation has gained acceptance and popularity worldwide in the medical community for its proven ability to help us handle our emotions better and support a healthy body.

Mindfulness meditation is getting a lot of attention in the press for its studied and proven health benefits. It turns out that mindfulness meditation not only helps us connect with our inner selves but also has extensive physiological health benefits. Neuroscientists have shown that mindfulness meditation does to the brain what exercise does to the body: It makes the brain stronger and more flexible.[1] Meditation is a tool to help us handle stress and many unpleasant feelings that arise in our lives. It can decrease stress, anxiety, addiction, depression, and eating disorders, and improve cognitive and immune functioning. Some studies have shown meditation's capability to reduce blood pressure, pain, cortisol levels, and even cellular inflammation.[2] Mindfulness meditation actually changes our brain by making new neuropathways and disrupting old ones. This has the profound ability to change the way we react and perceive the world—with decreasing stress and anxiety and increasing clarity. Scientists have also found that there is an increase in frontal lobe activity in the brain after meditation.[3] This frontal lobe activity cultivates an "approach state" which encourages people to confront a challenging external situation or internal mental function such as a thought, feeling, or memory.[3] Such "approach" states can be seen as the neural basis for resilience and can be a supportive function when making challenging lifestyle changes.

Mindfulness meditation is quite simple. First, find a seat on the floor, a firm chair, or some other space that is comfortable but supports alertness. With your eyes closed or partially open place your attention on breathing in and breathing out. It can be helpful to count your breaths to ten and then count backwards from ten to help you focus on breathing, but this isn't required. If your mind wanders simply let the thoughts go. Bring your attention back to your breath and start your count over again from one. You will notice how busy your mind can be with thoughts and stories—especially when emotions are high. Remember it is not a failure to find yourself thinking! The actual purpose of the meditation is to catch your thoughts and let them go in order to return to the breath. There is no right or wrong way to meditate so try to leave expectations out of your practice. Instead, try to find compassion for yourself regardless of how busy or still your mind is on any given day. You can perform this practice in as little as five minutes a day, and increase your practice to thirty or even sixty minutes a day if you feel inspired. The ultimate goal is to take this stillness practice of focusing on the present moment into your day-to-day life, so that during your daily activities you are more aware of your feelings, thoughts, and what is happening around you.

We have taught our young children mindfulness meditation through a game called "sitting still like a frog." We pretend we are frogs, and we sit still with our eyes closed and focus on our breathing. Every minute or so I will say there is a fly, and they will stick their tongues out to eat the fly, and then we go back to focusing on our breath and relaxing.

Personal Values

Connecting with personal values is another great way to deepen connection with your spirit. Values are those things that really matter to each of us, the ideas and beliefs we hold as special, such as family, spending time in nature, a strong work ethic, respect for others, etc. It is important to know and name our values so that we can remind ourselves how it is that we connect to our most authentic self. When we name—or even write down—our values, we have the ability to calibrate our day-to-day activities with these values. How do I choose to spend my time? Do my activities further my values? Do they detract from my values? Are they neutral? Performing this exercise helps us delineate what activities or decisions move us towards living our values and which prevent us from living our values. My husband, children, and I talk about our values as a family. At the beginning of each year, the values are written on a big white paper, which is then posted somewhere in the house. Seeing these written values periodically reminds us all to reflect on how well we are in touch with those values, and how our life decisions move us towards or away from them. For instance, when I see the value "focusing on the person I am with," I am reminded not to check my email while I am playing with my kids. Or when I read "spending time outdoors," I remember that it is worth the ten minutes it takes to get my kids' snow clothes on to go play outside.

Many people find that journaling really helps them connect to their values. I admit I have never been intuitively drawn to journaling, although I appreciate its benefits. Artist and bestselling author Julia Cameron discusses a form of journaling that has piqued my interest. Cameron, author of *The Artist's Way* and many other books on creativity and cultivating happiness, encourages a practice called "morning pages." Morning pages are a form of journaling first thing in the morning that give us the opportunity to connect with our spirit, have honest conversations about what is going on in our life, and to clarify our values. She suggests that it is important that we don't try too hard to *create* something on our morning pages and that instead we simply write down what pops into our mind. "I need to do the laundry today. I hate doing laundry; it never ends. I feel like a slave to my family sometimes. I just give and give and give to the point where I don't even know who I am anymore." We may find that we see patterns in behaviors, decisions, and feelings that we write about over time, and we are eventually called to listen to what our thoughts are trying to tell us. With this awareness, we can then choose to courageously take action to be more in alignment with our inner spirit, or not. When we give voice to our thoughts on paper, we have the opportunity to see our lives more clearly and can challenge ourselves to be honest about any divide between that which we value and how we are leading our lives. Our morning pages may actually give us inspiration—"I want to learn how to dance," or "I want to go back to school to become a nurse." It gives a voice to the yearning of our soul.

Cameron encourages readers to do this type of journaling in the morning because our subconscious is most clear and fresh at this time. She recommends writing three pages by hand every morning and guarantees that the process will have an impact on how we live a life more closely aligned to our essence and true potential. This may seem like a lot to do for many of us, as we reflect on what our mornings typically look and feel like. Start out with one page, or even three sentences, if that is less overwhelming. My first several morning pages sounded something like, "This is boring. Three pages is so long. I don't have time for this. What is the point of writing to myself? Am I at three pages yet? Maybe I should write bigger…" Seriously! I know that it is hard to carve time out for a practice like this when there is so much to accomplish during the morning hours. But throw yourself a bone and just do as much as you can, changing the writing amount to whatever will get your pen on the page. You may find the practice valuable and naturally create ways to accommodate it.[4]

Gratitude Practices

Expressing gratitude is one of the simplest ways to connect with our spirit and has been found to profoundly impact happiness, health, and connection with others. Put simply, gratitude is being aware of the blessings and abundance in our lives. When we can see the good (even in what we consider the bad) complaining becomes more difficult. The act of expressing gratitude immediately shifts our focus to what is abundant—and away from what is lacking. Remember, what we place our attention on grows. If we put our attention on what we are lacking we will likely develop our ability to be unsatisfied, unhappy, and grumpy. If we deliberately focus on expressing gratitude then we develop our ability to feel appreciation, to love others for what they do, and to feel grounded in the world being okay. Unfortunately, focusing on what we don't have is more intuitive or natural for many of us. Therefore, we develop practices to train ourselves to become grateful.

Practicing gratitude has been found to have several health benefits. For one, grateful people tend to take better care of themselves and engage in healthier lifestyle habits like regular exercise and a healthy diet. Gratitude has been shown to help us better manage stress and foster happiness. Grateful people also tend to be more optimistic, a characteristic that researchers connect to healthier immune systems. Gratitude strengthens relationships, creating opportunities for oxytocin release.

There are many ways to incorporate gratitude practices into your day.

- Notice your day-to-day world from a point of view of gratitude—you will be amazed at all of the things that we take for granted.
- A gratitude journal may also help you document one or more of the things you are grateful for each day.
- Try reframing the way you view people by shifting your focus from negative traits to positive ones. For instance, "The person with the awful odor at the gym," could instead be "The friendly person with a great smile at the gym."

- Set a goal of giving at least one compliment a day—either to a person or about the environment. For example, "I love the view outside of our back window; the mountains are gorgeous."
- Ask yourself what you can learn from bad situations.
- Practice not gossiping or criticizing for a period of time, such as ten days or a month.
- Say prayers of gratitude at meal time. Our family begins every dinner by holding hands and taking turns sharing our gratitude from the day. This immediately connects us to our spirits and each other, and focuses our minds on abundance rather than scarcity, before we dive into our nourishing meal.

The Inner Critic

Ironically we ourselves can be the biggest threat to connecting with our own spirit. Creating space to connect with ourselves and to know ourselves more deeply can be scary. Many of us have a fear of truly being known and seen by others and even by ourselves. This fear is subconscious and can be hard to recognize. We hide behind busyness and tasks to avoid having to deal with the vulnerability of our true self. We have negative inner dialogues that often make us feel "less than" or "not good enough." We struggle with trusting ourselves.

Interestingly, I have observed that there are times when I actually create my busyness as a result of these fears. I become busy, and even a little neurotic, when I am feeling unhealthy, scared, lost, or disconnected from myself. In the midst of these uncomfortable feelings I come up with tasks and activities to do so that I don't have to feel or focus on my emotional pain. The last thing I want to do in this unhealthy state is slow down and be with myself. What I end up doing instead is cleaning my house a thousand times over, organizing drawers, working long hours, or obsessing about school. I subconsciously create my own excuses to avoid slowing down. Ironically, I think I have an underlying fear that slowing down might call me to live a life that is more fully me. This is scary because it's possible that others may not like the true me. At times, I fear being too true to myself because if I am rejected or judged, or if I fail, then my fear of being unlovable or broken will be validated. Our subconscious self protects us because there is a lot on the line. I am protected on all angles when I fill up my day with busyness and don't allow time for true self-connection.

Have you ever paid attention to your internal dialogue? We all have an inner voice and to varying degrees we have a negative and oppressive voice that has been called the inner critic, negative self-talk, or self-criticism. This voice or inner dialogue can tell complete lies about who we are and what we can accomplish and it's sneaky enough for us to believe it. "Why would my spouse love me? I am ugly and rude. I am unintelligent. And, look at that double chin." Or, "What do I have to offer clients. Others are better than me, and I am not worth what they would have to pay me." When we talk to ourselves in this way we devalue our worth and negate the fact that we are at our very core perfect and good. If we take time to heighten our awareness of these negative thoughts, we may notice that they can be almost continual for many of us and that it is a repeating record of the same saga over and over. You'd think it would get old and that we would catch on sooner. Of course, a little self-criticism can help us reflect and improve how we interact with people and the world. But too much can lead to self-doubt, stress, and even depression. The inner critic pulls us away from wanting to connect with ourselves on a real level.

It is hard to want to slow down and be connected to yourself when there is a brawl going on in your own head. But it is precisely because it *is* so difficult that tending to your spirit by working with negative self-talk is absolutely fundamental. It wasn't until I was in my mid-twenties and in graduate school that I became aware of all the negative chatter flying around in my head. I can't believe that I didn't know about the wild party my thoughts were having before then. How could I be nearly thirty and not have noticed what was happening directly within me? The answer is simple: I wasn't taught about the inner critic and wasn't shown how to identify it or what to do about it.

The consequences of listening to the inner critic can be pretty severe. For me, when I listen to myself say, "You are unintelligent. Why are you even talking? Nobody cares what you have to say, and besides you can't even articulate yourself," I withdraw, retreat, hide and become small. I pull away from relationship and slip inside my internal cave to safety. The cave is safe, but it is suffocating. This is detrimental to my relationships. When I listen to myself say, "You would never be able to start a successful business. You don't know the first thing about marketing," I prevent myself from living my dream and doing something that I am passionate about. Instead, my self-protective side wants to play it safe in a job or role in which I don't have to risk failure in something that really matters to me. I end up starting to retreat from the world and even hide from myself. Whenever we believe the lies of the inner critic we feel small, inadequate, and disconnected from the truth of the greatness that we really are. These feelings of doubt then become a self-perpetuating cycle since they do not inspire us to spend quality time with ourselves. This "devil on our shoulder" needs to be placed in the light to remove its oppressive influence.

The following suggestions are ways in which to work with our inner critic to stop it from preventing us from living our dreams and causing us to retreat away from ourselves and others. Stopping the inner critic in its tracks allows us to better connect with our spirit and live the life we are meant to live.

Increased awareness: Start by increasing your awareness that the inner critic exists. Simply notice the negative chatter that is going on in your head. Be curious about it. Is there a pattern to the accusations of the critic? Do interactions with certain people make the voice louder or more present? How often does the critic come around? Then, open yourself to seeing the critic as separate from your true self and essence. Start to doubt, question, and reject the inner critic.

Put a character or name to the inner critic: We have many different types of critics and we can give them each a character. For instance, you might have a critic for body image, another for intelligence, and yet another for holy obligations. When I did this practice I immediately pictured

Donald Trump as the face of my negative thoughts towards my intelligence. When my negative inner dialogue comes up, I can picture Donald Trump, a round-faced grump with awful hair, furrowed brows, and an assaulting frown, spitting all over me as he tells me how awful and stupid I am. I can just look back at him with detached amazement at how bizarre and unreliable he is. I can then simply name his presence and see him off.

Calling out the critic: We can also work with our negative dialogue by questioning from a cognitive standpoint. We can stop and ask ourselves if our negative story or belief is really true. Byron Katie, bestselling author and founder of what she calls "The Work"—a system of identifying and questioning negative thought patterns—provides helpful steps for working with the inner-critic (as well as for working with negative thoughts about others). Her process is logic-based, and it takes you through four questions and then suggests you do a "turnaround." As an example, I will use the four questions of Katie's structure to work with the negative self-talk statement, *"I'm not a good mother."*

1. First, ask yourself if the statement is true? Is it true that I am not a good mother? It can feel pretty true to me that there are a lot better mothers out there, and I often find myself flailing. So maybe.

2. If you answer "yes" or "maybe" to number one, ask yourself, "Can I absolutely know that it's true?" If I ask myself this question related to my negative mother self-talk I think twice and say, "Okay, I can't absolutely know that I am not a good mother." So, my answer is "no" to this question, I can't absolutely know that it's true.

3. Next, ask yourself how you react, what happens, when you believe that thought? When I believe the thought that I am not a good mother I feel defeated, little, and discouraged. I don't feel inspired in parenting. I don't like having this belief.

4. After that, ask yourself who would you be without the thought? For me, without the thought that I am not a good mother, I would mother to the best of my ability and question myself less. I would feel inspired and proud of myself in my mothering abilities. I would focus on loving my family with confidence and being gentle with myself.

5. The last step is the turnaround. Find ways to make the statement opposite and identify two to three examples of how the turnaround is true. Turnaround: *I am a good mother?*

   How is this true?

   1. I spend time giving my kids one-on-one attention. I know they love that, and it is good for them.
   2. I try to feed them nourishing foods and limit unhealthy foods so that their bodies function optimally.
   3. I give them safety, security, and structure in hopes that they will thrive. I try to listen to their feelings and validate their experiences.[5]

When I finish this process, it is hard to feel so convicted in my original thought and story. Identifying truths to my turnaround allow me to loosen my belief in my negative storyline and see other truths—truths that actually inspire and motivate me. Through this practice, I become released from the repetitive, unhealthy story that I can blindly believe and get sucked into.

☑ LIVE IT. MODEL IT. TEACH IT.

LIVE IT.

☐ Find things that "connect" you most, whether it is church and bible study, meditation or yoga, walking in nature, reading self-improvement books, journaling, or another practice that you have learned. Only you know what helps you slow down and check in with your higher self.

- [ ] Prioritize time to slow down and connect with your spirit. This is the essence of self-care.

- [ ] Recognize times when you make excuses not to slow down. Explore if it is because you are afraid to face yourself.

- [ ] Consider experimenting with mindfulness meditation.

- [ ] Explore your personal values.

- [ ] Identify one gratitude practice that you can implement on a daily basis.

- [ ] Practice working with your inner critic and finding ways to catch negative self-talk and prevent it from destroying what is most meaningful to you.

MODEL IT.

- [ ] Our children watch how we live our lives and notice where we place our attention. It is powerful when they can witness what it looks like to "be" more and "do" less. In a culture full of movement and achievement it is invaluable for children to see the value of slowing down and creating the space to see and honor who we are inside.

- [ ] Set specific times to unplug from your phone, computer, and television, and allow your kids to see you in your spiritual element. Give them the gift of seeing what bliss looks like when we are *plugged-in* to our higher selves.

- [ ] Show your family what it looks like to have gratitude and to focus on the amazing, mysterious, abundant blessings, and positives in life.

- [ ] Talk positively about yourself so that your children have endless opportunities to see what self-love looks and sounds like.

- ☐ Demonstrate what it looks like to challenge your negative self-talk.

TEACH IT.

- ☐ Inform your family about the benefits of finding what it is that connects them to their spirit.

- ☐ Encourage your family to explore different ways to connect with their spirit. Your way might be church, but your child's way might be with a paintbrush or pencil. Help him explore different avenues and talk to him about what he feels and how he might know that he is connecting to his inner self.

- ☐ Help your children carve out "slowing down" time from their busy school, play, club, and sport schedules. It is important for them to have down time where they aren't doing, producing, or moving. We have quiet time at our house for one hour every day. The kids can nap, read, or put together a puzzle quietly and by themselves.

- ☐ Practice mindfulness meditation with your children. Make it fun like our "sitting still like a frog" practice.

- ☐ Teach your children about values and the importance in understanding personal values. As a family share your individual values and honor each other in your differences. Because values drive our decisions and behaviors, this is a great way for family members to understand why we all behave differently or have different views and priorities.

- ☐ Consider coming up with family values on an annual basis. It is important that these values come from every member of the family and reflect the whole of the family unit. Remember, values are what are most important to us on a deep level and help us to be more aligned with our spirit.

- [ ] Share the power of gratitude. Guide your children in regular practices of gratitude, whether at the dinner table, at bedtime, during holiday celebrations, or simple interactions throughout the day. Help them practice being aware of and verbalizing the things for which they are thankful.

- [ ] Teach your family about the inner critic. Help them give it a face and a name and experiment with language to help them disregard the negative thoughts that they have about themselves. My son has named his inner critic Bully Boy, and together we work to kick Bully Boy out of the picture because everything he says is a lie, and he is not wanted in our house.

- [ ] Teach your children the work of Byron Katie and create a simplified version for the little ones. This is a tool that they will be able to use throughout their lives to help them assess the validity of their thoughts and better understand their emotional responses, even beyond negative self-talk.

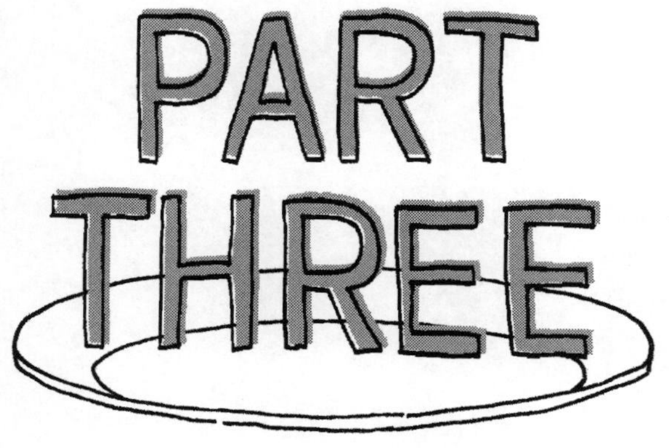

Secondary Foods

8

Real vs. Processed Food

The food that we consume has changed drastically over the last few decades and considerably so over the centuries. We eat nothing like our ancestors did. They ate food from the earth. We are now eating foods they would not even recognize, in amounts that exceed our caloric requirements, resulting in an epidemic of obesity and diabetes in people of all ages, including children. Chronic inflammation from the introduction and excess consumption of manufactured foods and refined sugars is a pervasive problem in our culture that is contributing to chronic disease and early death. Americans, and much of the world, are in a nutritional mess and, subsequently, a health crisis. The good news, however, is that this crisis can largely be addressed by changes to the food that we eat, and by getting back to the basic foods our ancestors ate not that long ago.[1]

It is becoming clearer that one of the biggest threats to American society is poor nutrition and fast food. Joe Cross, director and producer of the documentary *Fat, Sick, and Nearly Dead*, claims that the standard American diet kills seventy million people each year.[2] By eating healthier foods we have the opportunity to live longer, to avoid chronic illnesses like dementia, diabetes, and heart disease, and to drastically lower our odds of cancer.[3] The standard American diet, meals eaten by the average American, consists of about 60 percent processed food, 30 percent animal protein, 5 percent grains, and 5 percent vegetables and fruits. According to the U.S.D.A.'s "My Plate" food recommendations, Americans are advised to eat 50 percent vegetables and fruits, 25 percent protein, and 25 percent grains. Some nutritional experts claim that we should be eating 75 percent vegetables and fruits with the other 25 percent split between protein and whole grains.[4] Both of those recommendations shine a light on the huge gap between what we are actually eating and what we are encouraged to eat by health experts. It seems particularly noteworthy that none of the recommendations include processed foods. However, Americans are eating an exorbitant amount of processed and refined foods, and are nowhere close to getting enough of the foods that provide adequate nutrition and health (like vegetables and fruits). This is a major problem and a primary contributor to our current health crisis.

Our culture's eating habits are heavily influenced by convenience and emotional state. Clearly, in our "full plate" lifestyles we all look for quick and easy ways to feed our families. At the same time, many of us have developed patterns of eating based on emotional stressors. We may eat "comfort foods" habitually in order to cope with anxiety and depression. It is no wonder we find fast foods and convenient foods desirable. They are quick and usually taste good, filling our needs for convenience and comfort. But the reality is that the problems associated with most quick and convenient food have significant ramifications, as we are seeing in national health trends. The consequences of eating a highly processed, sugar-rich diet with few nutrients goes beyond being simply detrimental to our health. This diet is actually killing us. Yes, it is killing us! Many experts are pointing to our diet as the primary cause of most of the major causes of death in modern societies, including heart disease, cancer, diabetes, and Alzheimer's.[5] The Centers for Disease Control reported that in 2013 the U.S. had the highest obesity rates of the leading twenty-two industrialized countries. More than two thirds of Americans were reported to be overweight and one third of Americans were reported to be obese.[6] Childhood obesity is rising rapidly, more than doubling in children and quadrupling in adolescents in the past thirty years. Currently 18 percent of our children in this country are obese.[7] The rates of hypertension, Type 2 diabetes, heart disease, and other serious life threatening ailments are following similar trends. The connections between these patterns and diet will be explored in detail throughout Part Three.

Healthy foods are important to the developing bodies of our children. Did you know that the food we eat when we are young influences our health in adulthood? In addition to supporting our children's health to benefit them now, one of our most important roles as parents is to nourish our children's bodies while they are young to best set them up for good health and longevity when they are older. Nutritional deficiencies in younger years can create cellular damage resulting in serious illness (including cancer) in later life that can be difficult to resolve.[8] It's true that we cannot control everything that our children eat, and trying to micromanage their food could lead to emotional trauma resulting in eating disorders or rebellion against certain foods. That said, we do have the ability to choose what foods we keep in our home and define our family's eating values. These two factors will heavily influence the values and decisions that our children make outside of the home and when they are older. Kids will have to explore food for themselves and learn how eating well and eating poorly affects them, and we have to let them do that. In the meantime, though, we can establish a foundation that will serve them in their adult lives. At some point, they will blend the information they learned from early years with their own experiences. If children grow up eating primarily "real foods," this will surely have some influence on what seems appealing or right to them as they develop and discover their own strategy for health as adults.

Fundamentally, we need to shift our diet away from refined, processed, and manufactured foods and get back to eating "real foods." At the risk of over-simplifying, I am going to break all foods into two categories: "real foods" and "processed foods."

Real Foods

Real foods are those foods that are a product of nature and not of industry. The closer a food is to its natural state, the more nutrients it typically has and the more able our bodies are to recognize it as a nourishing substance. Our bodies know what to do with real food;

they thrive on real food. Michael Pollan, author of *The Omnivore's Dilemma* and other books on food-production trends, says that we shouldn't eat anything that our great grandmother wouldn't recognize as food. In other words, if our great grandmother wouldn't recognize a particular food, it is likely to be highly refined, processed, and/or manufactured. Some foods in the real food list below are processed minimally to allow them to be edible, like olive oil and other healthy fats, but the ingredients that make up the final product are all real and natural. Eating real food shouldn't be stressful or complicated; there are just a few things to understand and consider. The following are examples of "real foods" with short descriptions of their benefits:

Vegetables and fruits are perfect examples of real foods. Whether fresh or frozen, when you look at these foods you know what they are. Eating as many fruits and, especially, vegetables as you can handle is one of the best choices that you can make to shift eating habits. If possible, try to buy produce grown locally and in season. Our produce can travel half way around the globe before it makes it to our local supermarket and onto our plate. The closer to home we can purchase our produce, the more likely it is that it will hold higher nutritional value.

Be aware of processed products that claim to be vegetables, such as vegetable sticks, sweet potato chips, or dried pea snacks. Most of these snack foods have very few vegetables in them and are processed with unhealthy oils and added sugars that do not make them a healthy food or real food. Even though potatoes are a vegetable, we all know that potato chips are high in harmful fats and sugars, chemical preservatives, and addictive substances. Vegetable and fruit juices are similar: They typically contain very few vegetables and fruits and are high in sugar.

Dairy products like milk, plain yogurt, and cheese are considered real foods. Stick to products that do not have added sugar (avoid fruit yogurts) and are in their whole forms (like whole milk or raw milk). Reduced fat milk products usually have added sugar and additives to make them taste appealing.

When possible, purchase minimally pasteurized milk that is non-homogenized. Chapter 13 explores specific pros and cons of milk products.

Healthy fats like olive oil, unrefined coconut oil, avocado oil, grass-fed butter, and ghee are some examples of real food fats that provide essential nutrients to the body. Unfortunately, fat has gotten a bad rap. Contrary to what we've heard for the past thirty years, our bodies need fat, healthy fats, even saturated fats, and we should not cut such fats out of our diets. The low-fat diet fad of the 1990s has scared many people away from eating fats because they have been led to believe that eating fat makes them fat. It is important to understand that eating fat doesn't necessarily make us fat; sugar (which replaced all the fat in our previously yummy foods) is actually the primary culprit for causing fat in our bodies (because of its release of insulin—the hormone that allows fat to be stored).[9] Unfortunately, sugar is hidden in more foods than we often realize and is often a replacement for fat in "low-fat" foods. Our bodies rely on fat for optimal functioning. The goal is not to cut out all fats from our diet, it is to cut out the harmful fats (like trans-fats and polyunsaturated fats, described below).

Certified organic and grass-fed animal products are the healthiest choice if you eat animal products. The unhealthy and unnatural foods that are fed to conventionally raised animals impact the quality of the meat that ends up on our plates. If you have access to wild game, that is an optimal meat choice. Chapter 12 discusses the benefits of organic and grass-fed animal products.

Whole grains contain nutritious components but are commonly misunderstood, contributing to a significant problem in our typical diet. "Whole" grains contain the germ, endosperm, and bran. These various parts of the whole grain provide important nutrients as well as protect the body from absorbing the carbohydrate sugars from the grains into the blood stream too quickly. Common whole grains include whole wheat, oats, barley, maize, brown rice, rye, millet, quinoa, amaranth, and buckwheat. A refined grain like white rice or white flour contains only the endosperm. Be aware that the term "wheat flour" does not indicate whole wheat, but rather it is the same as refined white flour. These refined grains have been stripped of many important nutrients and cause spikes in blood sugar and insulin release which contribute to a host of inflammatory issues and diseases over time.

It is most nutritious to consume whole grains in their original form. When whole grains (even if containing the germ and bran) are turned into flour the grains absorb quickly into the blood stream and cause a spike in blood sugar levels, a problem that we will discuss further in the next chapter.[8] The germ and bran in whole grains slow the absorption of sugars into the bloodstream. Most packaged foods in the grocery store that claim to be whole grain or whole wheat (bread, crackers, pastas, etc.) are actually not in their whole form at all. They have had various parts of the grain removed and have been turned into flours. See Chapter 14 to learn more about grains.

Water is the best way to hydrate our body. We are made up of 50 to 75 percent water, and it makes sense that water should make up the majority of the liquids that we consume in a day. Drinking soda, fruit juices, vegetable juices, and sports drinks can be quite harmful to our health due to the levels of sugar they contain. Don't be fooled by clever marketing claiming that they benefit our health. One glass of orange juice (fresh squeezed or from concentrate) is equal to one can of soda from the perspective of increased blood sugar levels and the harmful effects to the liver and metabolism.[10]

Nuts and seeds are popular real food snacks in our house. Some nuts and seeds include walnuts, cashews, almonds, pecans, pumpkin seeds, sunflower seeds, and nut/seed butters.

Beware of granola bars and other packaged nut/seed products (including nut butters) as many of them are loaded with added sugars and harmful additives. See Chapter 9 to review the many names of sugar that can be hidden in these products.

All natural sweeteners including honey and 100 percent maple syrup are real food sweeteners; however, moderate consumption is advised since they still impact blood sugar levels and the release of insulin (which we will soon learn more about). Stevia is a good natural sweetener with zero calories and little effect on blood sugars and insulin.

Processed Foods

The following are examples of what I consider "processed foods." These foods are common in the American diet and can, in excessive amounts, be caustic to our health. I suggest that we limit these foods as much as we can. I'm not saying that we can't indulge every once in a while. The important point is that we recognize that the following foods are not supportive to health, and it is a good idea to eat such foods in limited quantities. We all need to find a balance that is realistic for ourselves. My husband avoids the following foods almost completely. I, on the other hand, am not so absolute, and I indulge in processed foods or refined sugars in limited amounts on occasion. We each get to decide what works best for us.

Refined grains such as white flour or white rice. Most whole wheat breads, pastas, and crackers are made from processed wheat which are similar in health risks to white flour. Savvy marketing makes us believe that we are buying whole grains when the food is actually highly refined and processed. Chapter 14 discusses some additional concerns about wheat and gluten products.

Refined sweeteners such as sugar, any form of corn syrup, brown rice syrup, or cane juice/sugar. Agave nectar has recently been marketed as a healthier, natural sweetener option, however in reality it has an even greater impact on blood-sugar levels than table sugar and high fructose corn syrup.[11] All refined sugar weakens our immune system, causes imbalances in our microbiome, and spikes insulin, all contributing to damaging inflammation and poor health. Chapter 9 highlights the grave health concerns caused by refined sugars and their overuse in our culture. Also steer clear of artificial sweeteners such as aspartame and sucralose. These alternatives are actually worse for our health than regular sugar; they affect blood sugar, are toxic, and are highly inflammatory.[12]

Most things out of a box, can, bag, bottle or package are usually highly processed and contain added salt, sugar, preservatives, and toxic dyes that lack any real nutrient density. When I purchase a packaged product, I read the ingredient list to make sure I recognize all of the foods on the list as real food and that there is no added sugar. Chapter 10 explains how to effectively read ingredient labels.

Polyunsaturated fats like safflower, sunflower, corn, soybean, cottonseed, sesame, and mixed vegetable oils are highly processed fats using extremely high heat and are often produced with chemicals. They contain high amounts of omega-6 fatty acids, which are consumed in excessive quantities in the standard American diet. Our bodies need a particular ratio of omega-3 and omega-6 fatty acids to be strong and balance inflammation. That ratio of omega-6 to omega-3 fatty acids should be around 2:1. The ratio for most Americans is more like 10-25:1, largely due to the over-consumption of processed foods that contain high amounts of polyunsaturated fats. Chapter 18 explains in detail the problems with omega-6 fatty acids causing inflammation.

Trans-fats are manufactured fats that were made to enhance the flavor, texture, and shelf-life of processed foods. They are also called "partially hydrogenated," "fractionated," or "hydrogenated" oils. Some common examples include shortening and margarine. Trans-fats are some of the most dangerous fats and cause tens of thousands of premature heart disease deaths each year.[13]

Genetically modified organisms (GMO) are foods whose seeds have been manipulated genetically to obtain certain characteristics in a plant. Scientists are now able to isolate specific genes and insert those genes into a food crop to produce particular desirable traits. These new genes might be introduced to produce higher yields, make crops more resistant to infection and pests, or even to enhance nutrients and vitamins in the crop. While these improvements are well intended, there are subsequent health and environmental concerns related to GMOs. One health-related theory posits that modifying the genes in our food makes the food difficult to digest in the body. The body identifies these foods as a foreign substance or a threat to the body and attacks them. Our body has a hard time recognizing GMO foods as real foods that it can use, rather than as foreign invaders from whom it needs protection. This attack causes internal inflammation.[14] In addition, GMO foods have proven to be a very real threat to the environment. They have caused an increase in pesticide use that has resulted in "super" weeds and insects that can only be killed with 2,4-D (an ingredient in Agent Orange).[15] As if the toxicity we are exposed to from that isn't enough, we are seeing changes in the Monarch Butterfly and bee populations that have been strongly linked to this increased use of pesticides.[16] By now, most of us have probably heard how crucial the bee population is to the earth's ecosystem and how the bee populations are struggling. The most widespread GMO foods are canola, corn (including high fructose corn syrup and corn syrup), soy, cotton, sugar beets, papaya, zuccini, yellow squash, and alfalfa. Look for labeling such as "non-GMO" or "organic" if you want to be certain that these foods have not been genetically modified. Organic labeling requires that products are non-GMO. Many developed nations do not consider GMOs safe. In more than sixty countries, there are significant restrictions or outright bans on the production and sale of GMOs. In the U.S., GMOs are in as much as 80 percent of conventionally processed foods.[17]

Fast food is generally highly processed and has harmful chemicals added to make it tasty and addicting. Even salads in fast food restaurants (and many popular chain restaurants) are often full of unhealthy additives to make them mouth-wateringly good.[18] Some salads have just as much unhealthy fats, sugar, and salt as a fast food burger, despite claims that they're a healthy option. It is possible to have healthy options when eating out at restaurants, but this will likely not be at a fast food or popular chain restaurant. Many smaller or local restaurants have healthy salad and vegetable selections. Do beware of the kids' menus at restaurants. Those selections are most often things like pre-made chicken nuggets, fries, and pasta made with white flour and unhealthy polyunsaturated and trans-fats. Instead, at restaurants pick real food items from the regular menu or share your meal with your children. Most often eating out is not going to be as healthy as the food that we cook in our own kitchens. When you do eat out, pick your restaurants wisely (avoid fast food and large chain restaurants), and like everything else, moderation is key—eat out as an exception, not as a rule.

☑ LIVE IT. MODEL IT. TEACH IT.

LIVE IT.

- ☐ Reflect on your eating habits and take note of what processed and real foods you currently consume.
- ☐ Decide what processed food habits you are ready to kick out the door and what real food habits you are open to welcoming into your lifestyle.
- ☐ Start slowly, pick one or two changes that you are able to implement.

- [ ] Commit to learning more about real foods and processed foods and experimenting with some changes.

MODEL IT.

- [ ] Your children will notice when you place attention on what you are putting into your body. If you are eating less fast food or buying more produce, they will see this. They will notice when you prioritize healthy foods and will more likely do so themselves.

TEACH IT.

- [ ] Talk about the difference between processed versus real food. You don't have to demonize processed food in order to make a point that it is not healthy and can have harmful effects. Put the majority of your attention on the benefits of real food.

- [ ] If you are up for it, involve your kids in cleaning out the cupboards to get rid of the highly processed foods that you have in your house.

9

The Top Two Eating Rules to Remember

There is so much information available about healthy eating. It's clearly on our minds. But have your ever noticed how contradictory the dietary advice we receive can be? One school of thought may advocate high amounts of animal proteins and fats for optimal health, while another will claim that eating these foods will lead to premature death. It is overwhelming to sort out the advice. However, despite the conflicting messages out there about what to eat and what not to eat, there are two basic rules that I believe are essential for any healthy eating plan. They are:

1. Limit refined sugar.
2. Increase vegetable intake, especially leafy greens.

Limit Refined Sugar

The media is full of stories about Americans' sugar addiction and the associated health consequences. Sugar has even been referred to as "the silent killer." That may sound dramatic, considering sugar has occurred naturally in the human diet for thousands of years. But the real problem today lies in the extreme overconsumption of sugar. The "fat-free" fad of the last few decades has resulted in foods being pumped full of various forms of sugar; companies had to find some way of making food taste good again once they took out all the fat. This has contributed to a dramatic increase in the overall consumption of sugar. But just how much sugar are Americans eating? Here are some sobering statistics about sugar consumption in the U.S.:

- In 1820, Americans consumed less than 5 pounds of sugar per year. Currently, each American on average consumes nearly 3 pounds of sugar each week and about 130 pounds of sugar per year. In a lifetime, we average 3,550 pounds of sugar consumption.

- In 1822, the average American ate 45 grams of sugar every five days—the equivalent of one twelve-ounce soda. In 2012, Americans consumed 765 grams of sugar every five days—the equivalent of nearly twenty twelve-ounce sodas.

- The American Heart Association recommends no more than nine and a half teaspoons of sugar per day—the equivalent of less than one can of soda. The average adult consumes twenty two teaspoons per day and the average child consumes thirty two teaspoons per day.[1]

The implications of such a significant change in sugar consumption over such a short period of time have been dramatic. Sugar is the primary dietary factor contributing to overweight and obesity, which in turn pose a major risk for type 2 diabetes, stroke, cancer, heart disease, hypertension, autoimmune disease, Alzheimer's, and many more life-threatening and life-limiting conditions.[2]

Don't be fooled into believing that these diseases only affect overweight people. Thin people can also be at great risk for some of these chronic diseases if they consume too much sugar. The term TOFI—thin-outside-fat-inside—is used to describe lean individuals with excess internal fat.[3] In other words, a thin person can have many of the same risk factors as someone who's overweight, due to poor health inside of the body. Thin does not equal healthy. Your level of sugar consumption is likely to be a better predictor of health than your waistline.

The Impact Sugar Has on the Body

Although we've been taught to believe that consuming fats is what makes us fat, sugar is by far the bigger culprit. This is bittersweet news. On one hand we can ease up on worrying about eating too much healthy fat, while on the other hand we are called to reduce our sugar consumption. I don't know about you, but I really enjoy sweet treats. As you read and integrate the following information on sugar, try not to be discouraged by thinking that you have to cut out every sweet treat from your life. For most of us, that would be an overwhelming endeavor. Rather, we each get to play with our eating decisions and determine the correct balance for ourselves. My mother, a self-proclaimed sugar addict, says that she has to stay away from refined sugar completely or she "falls off the wagon," finding herself knee deep in addictive behavior and continuing her cycle of on again off again weight gain and unhealthy eating habits. Conversely, I choose my sweets wisely. I don't buy meals and snacks with added sugar for our regular food consumption, and I limit refined grains and simple carbohydrates in our house. I do, however, enjoy a sweet treat every once in a while or for a special occasion. Moderation is key for me. I do know that I don't want to be wasting my "sugar allowance" on refined sugar that is hidden in my everyday foods. I want to save my sugar consumption for a fresh bagel or sweet treat at my favorite local bakery, for example.

One of the issues with sugar is that our bodies can only metabolize a certain amount, with the excess being stored as fat (especially in the abdomen). Up to one quarter of the calories that many Americans consume currently comes from added sugars.[4] This excessive consumption of sugar in any form (table sugar, honey, agave nectar, high fructose corn syrup, sucrose, dextrose, maltose, maltodextrin, etc.) triggers mechanisms in our body that lead to weight gain. Sugar is one of the primary foods that causes insulin releases. When we eat more sugar than our body can use for energy, insulin stores the excess as fat. The less insulin released, the less food is stored as fat. And the more insulin released, the more food is stored as fat. All forms of sugar—spanning from the obvious sweet treats to the starches in potatoes or the carbohydrates in grains—trigger this weight gain mechanism. The body reacts to sugar and simple carbohydrates very similarly. On the other hand, it takes significantly longer for the body to convert complex carbohydrates such as whole grains, beans, fruits, and vegetables into sugar. The longer the body takes to break a carbohydrate down into sugar the more regulated our blood-sugar levels will be. Regulated blood-sugar levels are better for both weight control and general health.[5]

In addition to causing weight gain, insulin released in high amounts over time leads to insulin resistance—the precursor to type 2 diabetes.[6] Despite my initial bad-mouthing, insulin is actually an essential hormone that helps us move sugar from our blood stream into cells where it can be used as energy. Whenever we eat carbohydrates (and to a significantly lesser degree when we eat proteins), the amount of sugar in our blood increases in correlation with the amount of sugar in the food. The pancreas releases insulin in order to help take the sugar out of the bloodstream and carry it to our organs so that it can be used for energy. The higher the sugar content in our food, the higher our blood-sugar level becomes and the more insulin is required to process the sugar. The rate at which a food raises blood-sugar levels is referred to as its glycemic index. The higher the glycemic index of a food, the more drastically it affects your blood-sugar level and the corresponding release of insulin. Habitually eating foods with a high glycemic index can make us less sensitive to insulin (or more "insulin resistant"). As we become resistant, our body has to produce more insulin in order to stabilize our blood sugar. Eventually the pancreas gets exhausted and stops releasing the hormone properly. Sugar gets stuck in the bloodstream, causing damage to the heart, nerves, and kidneys. This is referred to as type 2 diabetes, and individuals with this condition need to take a pharmaceutical form of insulin in order to transfer the sugar from their bloodstream to their cells. I mentioned earlier my mother's sugar addiction and her realization that she has to avoid sugar and simple carbohydrates completely. Because of years of carb abuse and excess sugar, she developed insulin resistance (pre-diabetes). She now understands that her body is at high risk for diabetes and other chronic illness, and she cannot afford to subject her body to any insulin bursts. In her pursuit to save her pancreas and her overall health, she successfully lost ninety pounds and has stabilized her weight for over ten years—just by paying attention to her intake of simple carbohydrates and sugar.

Insulin resistance doesn't just increase the risk of diabetes. In fact, some medical experts attest that insulin resistance is the most significant marker for a shorter lifespan.[7] Bursts of excessive insulin damages our body, ultimately leading to fatigue, joint pain, heart disease, a weakened immune system, and many chronic diseases associated with aging. It increases the risk of thyroid problems and several kinds of cancer.[8] Even high blood pressure is primarily linked to our body's overproduction of insulin. Over 85 percent of those with hypertension can normalize their blood pressure through simple lifestyle modifications, such as avoiding refined sugars and grains.[9] We have been so focused on cholesterol, fats, and salt in the fight against heart disease that most of us have not been aware of sugar's significant contribution.

On the path to developing the major health problems mentioned above, excess insulin first begins to manifest as more subtle symptoms. Initially, high insulin levels stimulate the production of pro-inflammatory chemicals called cytokines.[10] These chemicals result in inflammation at the cellular level, which can lead to major or minor physical discomfort (such as head and body aches, joint pain, and digestive issues), skin issues like acne, neurological conditions such as depression, anxiety, fatigue, difficulty paying attention, and weight gain that is difficult to reverse. Even more importantly, this inflammation is a precursor and major driver in the development of the more significant major chronic diseases.[11] Remember, this type of chronic inflammation can be subtle and imperceptible initially, manifesting over time as actual illness.

Although understanding some of these physiological processes can feel weighted, confusing, or just plain boring to many of us, understanding the basics of sugar's effect on my body has helped me make productive diet decisions. Recently while walking down the aisle of the grocery store, I spotted Reese's Peanut Butter Cups (in holiday shapes—my favorite). It was as if they were calling my name. My mouth started watering, and I fantasized about how that little morsel of goodness would melt in my mouth. My rational self quickly stepped in and pictured my blood sugar spiking, my pancreas working overtime to produce insulin, and I imagined the inflammation that would ensue as a result. Yes, this type of thinking may sound crazy and farfetched, but I think this way because I have become aware of the sugar-induced headaches or body aches that can follow such an indulgence. I ended up concluding that the temporary pleasure was not worth neither the potential immediate discomfort nor the long-term damage to my cells and body. I confidently (and sadly) pushed my cart on down the aisle.

The Many Places Sugar Hides

So how can we begin to reduce our sugar consumption without feeling deprived of this sweet, simple pleasure? Most of us are aware of the obvious sources of sugar, like candy, cakes, cookies, ice cream, and pies. These are often easier to limit or reduce because they are so obviously loaded with sugar. We tend to make a conscious decision to have them or not. In my opinion, though, the most dangerous sources of sugar are those that are hidden. Most processed food products, even items you would never guess, have some form of sugar additive—including some cheeses, milks, yogurts, breads, peanuts, frozen dinners, chips, bacon, spaghetti sauces, pickles, beef jerky, breakfast sausages, lunch meats, cereals, crackers, granola bars, condiments, bagels, salad dressings... The list is almost endless. But if we pay close attention to ingredient labels, we can identify brands that offer many of these same products without sugars and unhealthy additives (see Chapter 10). One challenge in particular is when food products are marketed as health foods with claims on the packaging telling us how they will reduce our risk of X, Y, or Z ailment. We often believe that we are eating something that is good for us, when in reality we are eating products that contain significant amounts of sugars and starches that are damaging to our health. We now know that refined sugar has no nutritional value and has been linked to a host of health conditions. But unfortunately, sugar is so pervasive in our modern food supply that we have to educate ourselves on where it can be hidden in order to avoid the most common illnesses of our day.

Soda and other sugared drinks, like sport drinks and fruit juices, are currently the largest source of sugar consumption in the U.S.— over one third of our total sugar intake. The average American drinks fifty-three gallons of soft drinks alone per year. Drinking soda, comprised primarily of high fructose corn syrup, is like injecting a shot of sugar right into the veins. This sugar spike triggers a drastic insulin release, which results in the calories from the sugar being quickly stored as fat, and over time leading to countless diseases. There have been some successful efforts to broadly reduce soda consumption—for example in many schools. But even as soda becomes less commonplace in middle and high schools, it has often been replaced by sports drinks, whose effects can be just as problematic. In fact, in 2012, sports drinks were still available to 83 percent of high school students and 55 percent of middle school students.[12]

Many people trying to make healthier choices are surprised to learn that fruit juice is no better than soda and sports drinks in terms of sugar content. Many of us believe that fruit juices are healthy because they are made from fruit. A more accurate name for fruit juice, though, would be "liquid fruit sugar." The majority of fruit juices on the market actually have sugar, corn syrup, or other sweeteners added to them. But even drinking pure fruit juice isn't the same as consuming the fruit itself. Whole fruit is full of fiber, which forces the body to digest the sugars more slowly than in the juiced form. When the fiber is removed, the juice that remains is a sugary drink similar to soda, which spikes blood-sugar levels and releases insulin in high doses. In fact, a cup of orange juice has nearly the same amount of sugar as a Coke.[13] One cup of white grape juice contains the same amount of sugar as four glazed Krispy Kreme doughnuts.[14] According to the U.S.D.A., increased consumption of juice, even 100-percent fruit juice, is associated with higher body weight in children. And adults who consume fruit juice on a daily basis have been shown to have higher blood pressure than those who do so only on occasion.[15] Many people drink fruit juice for a vitamin boost, but the fact is many vitamins available in whole fruit don't make it through the processing phase, which is why synthetic vitamins are so often added to the juice.

For many of us, our liquid sugar of choice comes in the form of a beer, cocktail, or glass of wine. As a culture, we consume a lot of sugar in our alcoholic drinks which can play a role in both weight gain and the development of chronic disease. Some find eliminating alcohol altogether a challenge, so weighing the options as they relate to sugar content can be helpful when making drink decisions. Wine generally contains low amounts of sugar; however, that is not the case for sweet wines. Some medium sweet wines have around thirty-five grams (roughly nine teaspoons) of sugar in the bottle. Sweeter wines have still more sugar. Stick with dry red and dry white wines if you are a wine drinker. Beer is low in sugar, but that is offset by its high amount of carbohydrates. A standard beer may contain no added sugar but have nearly twenty grams of carbohydrates. It is common for people who cut back on or eliminate beer to notice a dramatic difference in weight and wellness. Most distilled alcohols use sugar at some stage in their production; however, the distillation process often dissolves the sugar. The "clearer the better" when it comes to spirits and sugar. Vodka and gin are usually the lowest in carbohydrates. It is usually the added soda and juice mixers that are a bigger problem than the spirit itself. Try using club soda or mineral water as a mixer and adding lemon or lime for taste. Tonic water contributes about twenty-two grams (over five teaspoons) of sugar to your drink, so be careful not to confuse tonic water and soda water. The alcohol with the highest sugar content on its own is by far liqueurs (such as Kahlua and Bailey's). If you are looking to cut back on sugar intake, try to stay away from any cocktails containing these sugary mixers. Limiting or eliminating alcohol consumption may be an ideal health goal, but many of us aren't willing to make that lifestyle change. The next best thing is to cut back on the sugar content that we consume through our alcohol intake.[16]

Refined grains such as white and wheat flour are not technically sugar but rather simple carbohydrates that trigger the same reactions in the body as sugars. Chapter 14 discusses how grains that are made into flour are absorbed by the body similarly to sugar, resulting in high blood glucose levels. Products made with these flours have a high glycemic index, therefore, triggering insulin releases and leading to fat storage and inflammation. Examples of such food products include most breads, pretzels, crackers, bagels, cereals, and pizza dough, even when labeled as "whole wheat" and "multi-grain." Refined grain products should be treated with the same precautions as sugar.

With the awareness that consumption of large amounts of sugar can be unhealthy, some of us have made changes to reduce sugar use, such as buying sugar-free alternatives and diet sodas. But beware that sugar alternatives like aspartame (NutraSweet, Equal), sucralose (Splenda), saccharin (Sweet'N Low), and other sweeteners actually lead to some of the same problems as sugar itself, in addition to their own unique problems.[17] It has been shown that individuals who consume diet soda actually gain more weight than those who drink regular soda.

It isn't easy limiting sugar in our kids' diets. Sugar is everywhere—school lunches, birthday parties, friends' houses, classrooms and class parties, parades, holiday traditions, and celebrations. The list goes on. We can't always control what our kids eat, especially as they get older and more independent. But we can try to lay the groundwork by establishing boundaries with sweet treats, while at the same time educating them about the health consequences of consuming too much sugar. One example of a boundary we have set is our Halloween tradition. The kids choose five pieces of candy to eat and the rest goes into a bag for the Switch Witch. After bedtime, the Switch Witch replaces each child's candy bag with a special gift (coloring book, stuffed animal, small toy, etc.). For Christmas, Easter, and other holidays, we make homemade treats, give fruit, and buy goodies that are in alignment with our eating values, yet just as special as more typical holiday fare. If we are at a celebration, we attempt to teach our kids about moderation—having only one cookie, brownie, cupcake, etc. We send our kids to daycare with snacks if we think the snack options provided don't align with our dietary goals. Many parents I know make lunches for their kids every day for school, knowing that school lunches are typically high in sugar and refined grains. I try to educate my children—in terms they can understand—about what sugar does to their bodies. We talk about the difference between eating one and five pieces of candy in one sitting. Amazingly, I will often see them making decisions based on that understanding. They might save some candy for later, or they might ask an adult if a particular food is good for their body. I can tell they are making decisions based on our discussions.

Our Sugar Addiction

In addition to sugars hiding out in many of our favorite foods, we may also be increasing consumption because it is so addictive. Research using brain scans has found sugar to be as addictive as cocaine. Sugar has a powerful impact on the reward center of the brain called the nucleus accumbens; it causes a euphoric effect that triggers dopamine release (a chemical that controls pleasure in the brain). When we eat foods that contain a lot of sugar, a massive amount of dopamine is released in the brain. After continual over-consumption of sugar the brain adapts to increased dopamine levels, showing fewer dopamine receptors and more opioid receptors. This means that the next time we eat these foods, we need more to get the same effect. Therefore, sugar, junk foods, and, as you may have noticed, many of your favorites with hidden sugar are incredibly addicting. Their effect on the reward centers of the brain is similar to that of commonly abused drugs like cocaine, nicotine, and heroine. I am confident that I have an addiction to sugar based on how badly I can feel like I need a sugar fix. I have at times given in to the addiction and eaten my way through a whole box of cookies or bag of chips. It takes a concerted effort to keep my sugar intake in the moderate to low range. When I clear my body of sugar by totally eliminating it for a couple of weeks, I have a much easier time limiting my sugar going forward—I simply don't have the cravings. My experience is common. Many people who eliminate sugar from their diets initially experience withdrawal symptoms, such as headaches, anxiety, tremors, and even chattering teeth from the rapid drop in dopamine levels. It is truly a physiological addiction. We can't wait for our next sugar fix, and we need more of it to give us the feel-good sensation we crave. No wonder it is so hard to decrease our sugar intake.[18]

Unfortunately, many health care practitioners aren't aware of the profound influence that sugar has on most chronic disease. Developing an understanding of sugar and insulin's vast impact on our health is one of the most important steps you can take to optimize the health of your family. Avoiding refined grains, sugar (including soda, sports drinks, and fruit juice), as well as anything with high fructose corn syrup and artificial sweeteners will allow for more balanced insulin and blood sugar levels, minimizing the risks of multiple illnesses.

Increase Vegetable Intake, Especially Leafy Greens

The clichéd and somewhat annoying advice to eat your fruits and vegetables is far from news to any of us. We have heard it our entire lives. Yet, when asked if they would increase their fruits and vegetables if they knew that it was good for them, most people say they probably wouldn't. I think the importance of eating vegetables, and especially green leafy vegetables, is highly under-appreciated. Our naivety about the benefits of vegetables may stem from the indirect experience we have with our diet and its implications in our body. We may not notice the difference in our health condition from one day to the next as we eat, or do not eat, vegetables. Likewise we don't physically note the slowly developing damage caused by inflammation (from eating sugar-heavy and processed foods for instance). We only notice when it's too late. In other words, consequences down the road do not motivate us to eat vegetables today.

Veggie Resistance

I have to confess, that including enough vegetables in my family's diet is not natural for me. My taste buds prefer white starchy foods. I envy my husband who can eat a huge salad or a big pile of *any* vegetable on his plate and moan with satisfaction. I have to consciously remember to make vegetable dishes, and it's an effort for me to consume enough of these foods. My motivation to prepare vegetables for my family does not come from craving or loving vegetables, but rather from a place of rationale and awareness of their great health benefits. When I make a meal full of brightly colored vegetables, I internally cheer myself on by thinking, "Wow, I'm super awesome—look what amazing nutrients I'm feeding these lucky little dudes!" I have also learned to make really great tasting meals with vegetables and other delicious and healthy foods, but that doesn't make my love for the white foods just disappear. The more that I have learned about the detriments of sugar, starches, and processed foods, and the benefits of plant-based foods, the greater my commitment to providing as many vegetables as possible for my family. I know it is the right thing to do. My good friend has joked that when we were first getting to know each other and I was making salad for our two families for dinner one night, the bowl of salad I made was so small she thought to herself, "I hope she has a bowl for everyone else. What I've learned about veggies and their impact on our health has inspired me to push through my resistance—and I hope it will do the same for you.

I'm not the only American that has had a little resistance to vegetable consumption. We are a culture that, as a whole, eats too many processed foods and animal products, and not nearly enough plant-based foods. The typical American meal consists of a half plate of animal protein, a quarter plate of overcooked vegetables or white potatoes, and a quarter plate of white refined carbohydrate. Only about 5 percent of our total caloric intake comes from vegetables and fruits when it should be closer to 50 percent (some say 75 percent) of the plate.[19]

Veggie Revolution

Why are vegetables important in our diet? To begin with, vegetables are full of micronutrients. Micronutrients include vitamins, minerals, and antioxidants which are required for normal metabolism, growth, and physical well-being. Being deficient in these micronutrients has been linked with many common illnesses. Processed foods, on the other hand, contain mostly synthetic vitamins and minerals. With 60 percent of our diet coming from processed foods, many of us are lacking vitamins and minerals that our bodies need.[20] When foods are closest to their natural state, they contain higher volumes of vitamins and minerals, which the body can use more efficiently than synthetic nutrients. The best way to obtain all of our necessary daily vitamins and minerals is by eating a diet high in fresh fruits—and especially—vegetables.

Fruits, vegetables, grains, and legumes also contain phytonutrients, highly nutritious active compounds that protect plants from bugs, fungi, bacteria, viruses, and other threats, which in turn provide us with nutrients that prevent disease and help our bodies work properly. Eating sufficient vegetables and fruits ensures we have enough of these powerful agents to prevent major health conditions. You can think of phytonutrients as health boosters—not essential to keep us alive but necessary to keep us strong and healthy. We can appreciate the potential contribution of fruits and vegetables to our health when we consider that one orange contains more than 170 phytonutrients.

Phytonutrients come in many varieties. The list is long, but more common examples include carotenoids, flavonoids, resveratrol, glucosinolates, and sulfides. We probably know the most about carotenoids. Carotenoids are the phytonutrients that give fruits and vegetables their red, orange, and yellow colors. Phytonutrients are shown to help slow down the aging process and protect against a host of diseases, including some cancers, heart disease, high blood pressure, and other chronic health conditions.[16] They also have the ability to enhance immunity. (See Chapters 15 and 16 to learn more about the powerful role vegetables play in strengthening our immune system and protecting us against cancer.)[21]

In order to gain the greatest benefits from vegetables, aim for variety or "eat the colors of the rainbow." For instance, choose berries, tomatoes, orange and yellow fruits, and leafy greens. One rule of thumb is to try to eat at least seven different colored foods every day. Bright colors in vegetables often represent high levels of nutrient concentration—so, the brighter the better!

Cruciferous (cabbage-family) vegetables are highly valuable and will be discussed in relation to cancer in Chapter 16. These vegetables include: broccoli, cauliflower, cabbage, bok choy, and Brussels sprouts.

Green leafy vegetables are a vegetable family that we should really place great effort in making a part of our dietary habits due to their particularly powerful nutrients.[22] Did you know that green leafy vegetables truly are the "best thing since sliced bread?" Or maybe that saying should be, "the best thing to replace sliced bread!" This may come as a surprise since many Americans see green leafy foods as best reserved for rabbits, sheep, goats, and cows. But they are an excellent source of protein, can provide all of the body's required amino acids, are the best source of alkaline minerals, contain the best fiber, have many calming, anti-stress properties, and are the best source of chlorophyll.

Leafy greens include spinach, kale, beet greens, Swiss chard, lambsquarter, and the leaves of any other edible plant or weed (even dandelion greens!). For example, did you know that carrot tops have several times more nutrients than the actual carrot? And we usually throw that part away! The roots tend to taste better to us because they contain more sugar and water, but the real nutritional power is in the green tops. It is true that the tops of root vegetables and leafy greens in general can taste bitter due to the abundance of nutrients in them. But when prepared correctly that bitterness can easily be overcome, making leafy greens some of the most delicious dishes on the plate.

Victoria Boutenko, in her book *Green for Life: The Updated Classic on Green Smoothie Nutrition* suggests leafy greens should be in a separate category from vegetables, since they not only look different, but more importantly they also contain a completely different set of nutrients. Unfortunately, leafy greens can get overlooked in the "fruits and vegetables" category, even though their health benefits are both unique and profound.[23]

Let's take a look at one of the greatest health benefits of leafy greens—chlorophyll. Chlorophyll is responsible for the green pigmentation in plants. It absorbs energy from the sun to facilitate photosynthesis. Chlorophyll in plants is roughly equivalent to blood in humans. And not only is chlorophyll crucial to plants, it's also got some surprising benefits for humans:

- Serves as an antioxidant and anti-inflammatory
- Assists in growth and repair of tissue
- Neutralizes pollution that we breathe in everyday
- Delivers magnesium and helps the blood carry oxygen to all cells and tissues
- Assimilates calcium and other heavy minerals
- Stimulates red blood cells to improve oxygen supply
- Neutralizes free radicals that do damage to healthy cells
- Reduces bad breath, body odor, menstrual odors, and foul-smelling urine and stools
- Reduces the ability of carcinogens to bind with the DNA in different major organs in the body
- Contains anti-carcinogenic properties that may help protect against toxins.[24]

So while it's true that vegetables might not taste as mouth-wateringly good as fast food and processed foods, it must be noted that we train our taste buds, as well as our brains, with the foods that we routinely eat. Therefore, if we eat mostly processed, heavily salted, and sugared foods then those become the foods that will satisfy our taste buds. But if we eat a variety of fresh fruits and vegetables, our taste buds will learn to like those foods. So if we want to like vegetables, then it is important that we give our taste buds regular experiences with them. I often hear about kids who don't like many types of vegetables, and I believe that it is partly because they are simply unfamiliar with them. Some parents even say that their child just won't eat vegetables. All of us parents have probably been in the situation where we feed our child something, anything, just to be sure he has a full stomach. Who wants a hungry child waking you at night? But if we regularly offer processed or refined foods, we may be enabling the avoidance of vegetables. If a child doesn't like a vegetable the first time you offer it, don't give up. It is quite normal for adults and kids alike to need to try a food multiple times before beginning to like it. In the wise words of Elmo, "If at first you don't like it, try try again." Frequently offering a wide variety of vegetables will help children learn to enjoy them over the long term.

Many people claim that they lack the will power to avoid comfort foods. They say that salads and vegetables are tasteless. They give excuses for their poor eating habits by talking about quality of life and enjoying the years they have with food they love. As with many things in life, I think we tend to focus too much on the short-term benefits of our experiences, often at the expense of our long-term experience. As I have learned about the impact of diet, and consumption of vegetables in particular, on our health as we age, I have begun to look at quality of life as much more than just loving what touches my palate. Quality of life is feeling physically well and able to participate in life—now and later, being free from debilitating diseases, living a long and full life, and being able to engage with mental clarity in the things that matter most.

It is no secret and no lie that we feel better when we are in better health. But it can be surprising just how great an impact eating enough vegetables and leafy greens—as well as limiting sugar—can have on our health and on bringing about all of these desired long-term outcomes. This insight is what motivates me to regularly provide a variety of vegetables for my family. When our bodies are well, we can often cure our own ailments and live longer lives. Eating vegetables can be the first step towards true quality of life, now and in the long term. And the good news is there are plenty of blogs, cookbooks, e-books, web-based meal-planning programs, and other sources that are full of tasty, healthy vegetable dishes that can make eating vegetables exciting. Eating healthy does not have to be bland and torturous!

My family makes sure to get green leafy vegetables into our diet starting immediately with breakfast, when we all drink at least one green smoothie. A green smoothie is a combination of a whole lot of leafy greens blended with some fruit and other goodies (like coconut milk, flax seed, chia seed, cacao, avocado, cinnamon, etc.). We call these liquid powerhouse drinks "ninja juice" in our house. The boys drink them up as they flex their muscles and talk about how fast their bodies are growing as a result of the juice. This is also a great way for someone like me to get a punch of vegetables early on in the day when I might not naturally think to add vegetables to my breakfast. My husband loves how he feels starting the day with ninja juice so much that he takes a small high speed blender on all of his work trips. We also eat kale salad almost daily and my husband is a master at sautéing Swiss chard in the mornings for breakfast. Through repetition, our boys have developed a palate for not just vegetables but for green leafy vegetables. Just recently my middle son told his dad after an ice skating outing that he was "hungry for something with chlorophyll." And when Santa asked the boys what their favorite foods were, my oldest son said "spinach," and my younger two sons both said "broccoli." We never stopped offering our children vegetables, even after those initial rejections. Now I feel grateful that my kids have developed their taste buds to enjoy healthy vegetables and reap the lifelong benefits they will provide.

☑ LIVE IT. MODEL IT. TEACH IT.

LIVE IT.

- ☐ If you're up for it, completely eliminate sugar for at least two to three weeks to clear your system of sugar dependence.

- ☐ Challenge yourself to significantly decrease your sugar intake. You will notice a huge difference in your energy level, mood, and general health.

- ☐ Experiment with adding more vegetables to your diet. Start with baby steps, but keep in mind that to optimize health 50 to 75 percent of our diet should consist of vegetables.

- ☐ Buy a vegetable that you have never cooked and learn how to prepare it. Try new recipes. The more vegetables that you are comfortable cooking, the greater the variety you will eat and the more your taste buds with get accustomed to new flavors. Vegetables are your friend, so begin to explore and get friendly with the many different types.

- [ ] Try not to focus on the list of foods you "can't have." Focus on the many amazing foods that fuel your body and that you know are supporting your health.

MODEL IT.

- [ ] Your kids will notice when you stop reaching for sweet treats or highly sugared products during stress or when processed sweet treats are removed from the cupboards. When you start drinking water or grabbing nuts or vegetables to curb your cravings, they will watch and learn these healthy habits for themselves.

- [ ] When your kids see your excitement about trying new vegetables or experimenting with foods that are new, they too will start to see vegetables through a new lens. When you start to enjoy vegetables, they will naturally become curious.

- [ ] Model bravery by trying unfamiliar vegetables multiple times as a way to train your taste buds to like a greater variety of foods. Show your kids you will try foods again if you don't initially like them.

TEACH IT.

- [ ] Don't be afraid to talk to your children about the many consequences of sugar in our body. Explain what happens to their blood sugars and how insulin is released in high amounts to get the sugar out of their blood. We talk about blood sugar with our small children often—using language that they can relate to.

- [ ] Inform your family about the many benefits of vegetables. We talk a lot about vegetables and all of the nutrients in the fresh food that we cook or prepare. We talk about the bright colors and the vitamins that help us feel strong and healthy. My kids love picking out things with chlorophyll and telling guests how healthy chlorophyll is for the body.

10
Reading Food Labels

I haven't always been a food-label junky. Ten or so years ago I didn't pay attention to the ingredients in the food I ate. I may have glanced over the nutrition facts to see how much sodium or fat was in a product, and I still probably didn't know what that really meant. However, I have learned how important it is to know what ingredients are in the food that I am purchasing for my family, and I now look at every single label on a product before I purchase it (if it has a label, which I prefer it doesn't because fresh food needs no label).

I have also encouraged my children to be involved in this endeavor by asking them to pick out items off shelves and review the ingredients to help me pick out the best ones. For example, I have asked my kids to pick out peanut butter that they want to buy. We read through the ingredients together and decide which one has the healthiest ingredients. In our grocery store, there is only one peanut butter brand that does not contain added sugar or a corn-syrup product, and my kids know that we do not buy foods with sugar unless we decide we are buying a treat for a special occasion. Now they know what brand we buy and are eager to pick it out with pride. I think it is important that our children see us reading labels and assist us in determining what the good, the bad, and the ugly are in the ingredient lists.

Here are the rules that I go by when I am reading ingredient labels and determining what to feed my family:

No sugar! If there is any sugar listed in the ingredient label, I will rarely purchase it. To me sugar in an ingredient label is a sign that the product is likely highly processed, and in our country's already highly sugared diet any extra sugar is worth staying away from (see Chapter 9). When you start to look, you will likely be amazed at how many food products contain added sugar, even foods that have savvy marketing claims trying to convince you that they are nutritious or "natural." We can only avoid sugar if we know all of its disguises and know what to look for. The following ingredients are all forms of sugar or substances that the body metabolizes just like sugar and should generally be treated as "code names" for added sugar:

The many names of SUGAR

- Sugar
- Corn syrup
- Cornstarch
- High fructose corn syrup
- Brown rice syrup
- Brown sugar
- Crystaline fructose
- Dates
- Ethyl maltol
- Fructose
- Fruit juice concentrates
- Honey
- Malt syrup
- Raw sugar
- Oat syrup
- Rice syrup
- Sucrose
- Turbinado sugar
- Cane sugar
- Molasses
- Agave nectar
- Barley malt
- Beet sugar
- Cane juice
- Evaporated cane juice
- Caramel
- Carob syrup
- Glucose
- Galactose
- Maltodextrin
- Maple syrup
- Confectioners sugar
- Rice bran syrup
- Tapioca syrup
- Potato starch

I may cook or bake with honey, dates, maple syrup, or coconut crystals for a special occasion, but as a general rule I rarely buy foods that have even those natural sweeteners listed in their ingredients. Even though some natural sweeteners have benefits—raw honey is known to have many health and medicinal uses—the body still experiences them as sugar in the blood stream that causes spikes in insulin. I use natural sweeteners in my own cooking and baking at home, but I am conscious of the amount that I add. I assume that store-bought food with these natural sweeteners in them are sweetened more than I would choose in my own kitchen.

I also avoid purchasing products that have artificial sweeteners in the ingredient listing, which may be as bad or worse for our bodies than sugar. Some common artificial sweeteners include aspartame, saccharin, and sucralose.

Avoid the unpronounceable! Whole foods are typically easy to recognize and pronounce. Chemicals, dyes, and preservatives tend to have long names that are hard to pronounce and often unrecognizable. If it takes you a couple of seconds to sound out a word or you don't recognize what it is, most likely you should stay away from it.

Limit/avoid safflower, sunflower, soybean, corn, cottonseed, and mixed vegetable oils. These oils contribute to oxidation and free radical damage, processes that lead to cell damage. These fats are so unstable they are vulnerable to damage from heat, making them rancid during the cooking process. However, they continue to be the main choice for restaurants and fast food because they are cheap. These oils are also high in omega-6 fats, which can lead to inflammation (chronic and unproductive inflammation!).

Look for whole grains. If your family eats grains, ensure the food you purchase contains the whole grain. I recommend that you reduce your consumption of foods made with flour, even whole wheat flour, and especially store-bought bread and most packaged snack foods (including chips and pretzels). Whole wheat flour has roughly the same glycemic index as white flour.[1] Both whole wheat flour and white flour cause spikes in blood sugar that can be even higher than plain table sugar. It is very hard to get any true whole grains in most store-bought breads.

There are some sprouted whole wheat breads that are closer to a whole grain product (such as Ezekiel brand sprouted bread), but I have never seen whole grain bread in the dry aisle of a grocery store that is legitimately whole grain. Be aware that "wheat flour" is another name for white flour. "Whole wheat flour," on the other hand, is different than white/wheat flour. It is a more whole form of the wheat germ, however, it is still pulverized and destroyed in the modern flour-making process.[2] If you choose to eat grains, try to eat them in their whole form, where the grain is intact or simply cracked into a few large pieces, such as with brown rice, quinoa, millet, and bulgur wheat.

No partially hydrogenated oils. Partially hydrogenated oils are a kind of trans-fat. Trans-fats are formed when manufacturers turn liquid oils into solid fats, such as margarine and shortening. Partially hydrogenated oils are used by food manufacturers to improve the texture, shelf life, and flavor stability of foods. Trans-fats contribute to an increase in and oxidation of LDL (low-density lipoprotein) cholesterol, which contributes to heart disease and inflammation in the arteries, and has recently been linked to Alzheimer's disease.[3] We can't just look at the nutritional labels on foods to ensure that there are no trans-fats. We must look at the ingredient list to see if partially hydrogenated ingredients are listed. If the amount of trans-fats are small enough per serving size, they can actually say 0 grams trans-fat on the nutrition label. A good rule of thumb is to stick with the real deal, like real butter, as opposed to the imitation product.

Focus on real food ingredients! I like to see that my ingredients are derived from real vegetables, fruits, herbs, and spices. It is important to me that I recognize the foods that are listed in the ingredients, as fruits and vegetables in particular.

The following ingredient lists from actual food products in my grocery store demonstrate why it is important to look at labels on everything we buy. Each brand has a unique twist on what it includes in its ingredients. Notice that the ingredients in simple, common food products can vary greatly by brand. The ingredient list in the middle column meets my real food standards and the list in the right hand column is its processed food nemesis, full of sugars, preservatives, and other ingredients. I am often shocked by the different ingredient lists I encounter in the store.

Product	Real Foods- In My Cart	Processed Foods- Back On the Shelf
Peanut Butter	Peanuts	Roasted peanuts, sugar, molasses, fully hydrogenated vegetable oils, mono- and diglycerides, salt.
Peanuts	Peanuts	Peanuts, sea salt, spices, dried onion, dried garlic, paprika, natural flavor, sugar, gelatin, torula yeast, cornstarch, dried corn syrup, maltodextrin.
Spaghetti Sauce	Organic diced tomatoes, water, tomato paste, organic extra virgin olive oil, organic roasted garlic puree, sea salt, organic hydrated onions, organic vinegar, organic garlic powder, organic spice.	Tomato paste, water, diced tomatoes, tomatoes, tomato juice, citric acid, calcium chloride, sugar, dehydrated garlic, canola oil, salt, onion powder, spices, sea salt, citric acid, parsley flakes.
Shredded Cheddar Cheese	Organic cultured pasteurized part skim milk, salt, enzymes, cellulose	Pasteurized milk, cheese culture, salt, enzymes, annatto (vegetable color), potato starch, corn starch, calcium sulfate.

Reading labels is a foundational tool when choosing foods to purchase. If you're not already doing this, my challenge to you is to read the label of every product that you purchase. It may take a little while to build confidence in knowing what is healthy and unhealthy, but forming the habit is a very important first step. Allow time to explore, look up, and inquire about the many different ingredients that make up the food you feed your family. A good general rule is: the fewer ingredients, the better. Take note that the listed ingredients on a food label are in descending order of predominance by weight—in other words, the list goes from most prevalent to least.

The Myths in Marketing

We can't totally blame consumers for choosing the sugary, highly processed foods that make us fat and sick. Food marketing schemes have us duped, making millions off of our naivety and blind trust. We read the front of a box or container and easily believe that the "low fat," "gluten free," or "low calorie" claim means that it is healthy for us. Why wouldn't we trust these claims about food? Aren't health claims on food and drugs regulated by government rules? The reality is that food marketers have developed highly effective buzz words that lure us into purchasing a supposedly healthy item that may actually be harmful and cause disease.

For example, I have yet to find a cold breakfast cereal that I would consider truly beneficial and healthy, yet marketing efforts have even convinced us that sugary cereals are healthy because they are "gluten-free" or "heart healthy," despite being loaded with sugars and refined grains. Standard granola bars that are full of many forms of sugar claim that they are natural and a perfect protein snack. During the low-fat fad of the 1990s, food companies started developing and promoting "low-fat" products. Companies were replacing fats with sugars so they would still taste good. What we didn't realize was that "high sugar" is a poor replacement for the harmful "hydrogenated fats" that we were trying to replace. Put simply, we replaced one unhealthy ingredient with another.

When I see the following claims I am automatically suspicious and always further investigate by reading the ingredients before I purchase.

"Low-Fat"— Usually means sugar and preservatives added to preserve taste.

"Fat-Free"—Usually means sugar and preservatives added to preserve taste.

"Multi-Grain"—Misleading buzzword; these products are often no better than those products made with refined grains, like white flour, when it comes to blood sugar and insulin.

"Natural"—If a product claims to be natural, it means that it wasn't made from artificial ingredients. Sugar, high-fructose corn syrup, and white flour are all derived from natural ingredients and, therefore, are included within the term "natural," despite being highly refined and harmful to our health. There are no regulations on the term "natural."

"Organic"—It is true that organic confirms certain standards over conventional products; however, being "organic" in and of itself does not ensure that the product is healthy. There is a lot of organic junk food out there, like organic cookies, organic ice cream, and organic candy. Being organic only speaks to how a product is grown or raised. It doesn't say anything about the nature of the product—for example, organic sugar. Even if the package says organic it is still important to read the ingredients. See chapter 12 for more information on organic practices.

"No High-Fructose Corn Syrup"—Although it's true that avoiding HFCS is important, check to see that other sugars have not been added in its place.

"Heart Healthy" or "Lowers Cholesterol"—It is often misleading and unfounded. When you see this marketing claim, review the ingredient label and make your own judgment about the product. If you want heart healthy foods, find the produce aisle.

"Gluten-Free"—Most processed "gluten-free" products replace gluten with starchy substitutes and often contain high amounts of added sugars, making these products hard on blood-sugar levels and insulin release. For healthy gluten-free options, shop the produce aisle or make products at home with trusted ingredients.

The outrageous and misleading claims that we find on so many food products are frustrating—especially considering the efforts that many of us make to be healthy. These health claims, in fact, may be a major contributor to the illness epidemic we find ourselves in. In my opinion, these misleading claims are unethical, if not criminal. Unfortunately, we must not blindly trust any health claims on packaged/processed food but rather question, doubt, and inquire further about the quality of the food for ourselves. Begin by reading the ingredient labels on every item that you put into your cart, no exceptions, and you will find yourself miles ahead of the game!

☑ LIVE IT. MODEL IT. TEACH IT.

LIVE IT.

- ☐ Challenge yourself to read every label before you decide to buy food products.

- ☐ Be suspicious of sneaky marketing tactics that attempt to convince us the food we are purchasing is healthy.

- ☐ Learn about the ingredients that aren't familiar to you. Even if you continue to buy processed foods as you ease into lifestyle changes, at least read the labels to build your awareness of what you are eating.

MODEL IT.

- ☐ Kids watch everything we do, including how we shop. Most of us have a budget for how much we can spend on groceries. It is a balancing act to find the best value within the realm of purchasing quality food. I try to find the most cost-effective product that also meets our eating values and food guidelines. For example, I choose the grocery store brand organic spaghetti sauce with real ingredients that is four dollars versus the nine dollar fancy spaghetti sauce that has real ingredients. Or, if organic cauliflower is eight dollars, I will choose the cheaper non-organic (knowing cauliflower typically doesn't have a lot of pesticides). When your kids watch you read labels and choose your foods based not on price alone but also on the value of the nutrients in the food, they too will learn that balanced way of shopping.

- ☐ Show your family what it looks like to trust the ingredients on the back label over the fancy and catchy, yet deceptive marketing claims that catch our eye. Demonstrate to your children that selecting quality food products is important, even when we feel rushed and less than completely informed.

TEACH IT.

- ☐ Show your children what to look for on ingredient labels. If they can't read, you can still read them the ingredients and make it fun. If it is a long word you have never heard of, make it sound silly and say something like, "I don't want that silly chemical in my body. Ewwwy." Have them help you pick out foods and look at the ingredients together.

- ☐ If you don't believe the ingredients meet the real food rules, then tell your children that you only buy foods that nourish their bodies, and your money isn't going to buy things that are harmful. If you choose to have a special treat or a food you typically wouldn't buy, talk about when that is appropriate and why. Sometimes we eat refined and processed food, and that is okay on certain occasions.

- ☐ Teach your family about savvy marketing that is designed to trick them. Pick up a box of cereal and say, "Now isn't this interesting.

This box of cereal says that it is low-fat and is heart healthy. When I look at the ingredients, I see that it has a lot of sugar and many processed ingredients. They can't trick me with that sneaky marketing."

11

How Our Microbiome Controls Our Health

Did you know that there are ten times more bacteria than cells in your body? That's right. Our bodies are complex ecosystems made up of more than one hundred trillion microbes.[1] These microbes make up 90 percent of our cells, leaving only 10 percent as "human" cells.[2] Some experts in this field claim we are actually more of a host than we are an individual being. That may sound creepy, but the reality is that these bacteria, fungi, protozoa, and even viruses are essential for our immunity, health, and nutrition. Like any complex ecosystem, these microbes must be balanced and cared for in order to be healthy. This system of microbes that live in our mouth, nose, throat, lungs, gut, urogenital tract, and on our skin is known as the "human microbiome," also referred to as microflora in this chapter.

Basically, within every anatomical niche of our bodies resides a complex, specialized group of microorganisms that serve us in many ways. The term microbiome was coined by Joshua Lederberg, an American molecular biologist, who argued that the microorganisms of bacteria, fungus, and protozoa inhabiting our bodies are extremely important when talking about both health and disease.[3] A better understanding of this complex internal ecosystem provides us with a vast, new source of healing potential. The nature and make-up of the microbiome varies from person to person based on factors such as diet, health history, ancestry, and even geographic location. But for all of us it is critical to understand the role that the microbiome system plays in maintaining (or not maintaining) our health.

This subject is near and dear to my heart. Our middle son had physiological and behavioral challenges for the first year and a half of his life that were perplexing to us and dismissed by his medical team. We eventually found medical doctors and naturopaths versed in the significance of the microbiome, who taught us a lot about the impact of our intestinal microflora on health. Through physical assessments and labs, my son was diagnosed with a yeast and bacterial overgrowth in his gut that was causing poor digestion, poor nutrition absorption, abdominal discomfort, loose stools (he didn't have a solid bowel movement in his first eighteen months of life), anxiety, poor sleep, and irritability. Prior to this, we didn't realize that his behavioral challenges could be a result of the health of his digestive system (which hosts his intestinal flora). We were subsequently able to treat the yeast and bacteria overgrowth, while supporting the growth of beneficial microbes, and his symptoms diminished significantly. Because his gut was so inflamed and damaged by the overgrowth, we continue to heal his digestive system by nourishing it with beneficial foods, avoiding certain foods that we know cause inflammation for him, and "feed" his good microbes with probiotic supplements and fermented foods. These interventions will be discussed later in this chapter.

As we have learned through our son's experience, the normal intestinal microbiome serves several purposes including protection against pathogen invasion, development of the immune system, and optimizing nutrition. I was thrilled to learn that we have so many little gut friends advocating for our health. But beware, as there can also be some bad guys mixed in with this gut flora who are believed to play a role in the development of inflammation, obesity, and many chronic diseases. My son had an overgrowth of these bad guys, and it was evident to us that the inflammation in his body was causing him discomfort and anguish.

To support our own good flora and ward off the bad flora, we first need to understand how our lifestyle choices nurture one side or the other. The highest concentration of our microbes hangs out in our gut, supporting our immune system, protecting us from disease, detoxifying our bodies, and even keeping our weight balanced. But unfortunately for many of us, our microbiome is becoming increasingly unbalanced or "dysbiotic," and this imbalance is being shown through science and research to be a significant cause of illness and disease. Dysbiosis can weaken immunity and lower dopamine and serotonin levels, causing mood instability. It contributes to nutritional deficiencies, lower thyroid functioning, increased cortisol releases leading to fatigue and ultimately causing inflammation and oxidative stress (the damage to cells from free radicals). Dysbiosis also causes "leaky gut syndrome," or a damaged bowel lining, which allows toxins, microbes, and undigested food to leak out of the gut, resulting in an immune response—which impacts the body both locally and systemically. Additionally, it contributes to increased hunger from increases in the hormone ghrelin and decrease in the hormone leptin, which of course leads to weight gain. Although physically located in greatest density in our gastrointestinal tract, this flora is in many ways responsible for controlling the health of our entire body.[4]

Awareness and research about the human microbiome, and the links between illness and dysbiosis as significant determinates of our health, is growing, although it is still a topic that is not typically discussed in conventional medicine. As with many of the lifestyle and diet factors covered in this book, dysbiosis has a direct link to inflammation and all of its ramifications. In fact, dysbiosis and inflammation have a unique relationship in that they feed each other. Dysbiosis causes inflammation, and inflammation contributes to dysbiosis. The compounding effect of this relationship may result in exacerbated or accelerated development of the following conditions:

- Allergies
- Autoimmune disease
- Obesity and type 2 diabetes
- Colorectal cancer
- Infant immune deficits
- "Colic" in infants
- Asthma
- Food sensitivities
- Mental illness (for example depression, anxiety, bipolar symptoms)

- *Behavioral problems (for example, Attention Deficit Hyperactive Disorder, autism, Attention Deficit Disorder)*[5]

Because there are often, but not always, bowel-related issues associated with dysbiosis, many individuals with dysbiosis are diagnosed with Irritable Bowel Syndrome (IBS), which tends to be a conventional diagnosis for "irregular bowel patterns of unknown cause." According to the naturopaths and medical doctors that helped us with our son, the underlying problem in many people with IBS is an unbalanced microbiome.

My son was initially given a "probable diagnosis" of IBS from a pediatrician, due to his irregular and abnormal bowel patterns. After we sought a second opinion that guided us towards eradicating problematic bacteria and yeast in his gut and supporting healthy intestinal flora, his bowels were the first thing to normalize. Before receiving this insight, we also had speculated about other traditional diagnoses for him. There were moments when I wondered if he was on the spectrum of autism because of his behavioral outbursts and inability to regulate his emotions. Thankfully, once his gut became balanced his emotional and psychological struggles dissipated as well. Thank goodness that we were led to the root cause of these challenging and uncomfortable symptoms rather than continuing along a path that could have led to medication-based strategies—and potentially feeding the problem unknowingly through continued damaging lifestyle habits.

Microbiome Mishaps

There are several factors that can cause disturbances in, or alter the bacterial composition of, our microbiome. There have been drastic changes in the typical American microbiome in the last forty years due to the following reasons:

1. Increase in Processed and Manufactured Foods

Our modern industrial food sources stimulate different organisms in the gut than do natural, real foods. The foods that we know are required to feed a healthy microbiome are no longer common in the average American diet. Other foods can damage the healthy microbes. Topping the list of microbe-killers are processed foods, genetically modified organisms, sugar (especially high-fructose corn syrup), and wheat. Studies have revealed a positive-feedback loop between the foods we crave and the composition of our microbiome, which depends on those nutrients for survival. So if you're craving sugar and refined carbohydrates, you may actually be feeding a voracious army of Candida (a type of yeast). Sugar feeds both harmful yeasts and bacteria in the microbiome, throwing off our healthy balance and causing widespread malfunctioning in the body. This imbalance is common in America because of the high amounts of sugar we consume. Agricultural chemicals such as herbicides and pesticides are other common offenders. These chemicals, designed to kill plants, bugs, and pests to protect our food, have been shown to also attack our friendly flora. Multiple recent studies have shown that one of the most widespread herbicides used in modern agriculture suppresses the growth of our good bacteria and leads to the growth of harmful bacteria.

2. Increased Exposure to Antibiotics

In our current medical system, antibiotics are frequently offered as a standard treatment for many infections, even though it has been found that they are needed in only about 10 percent of the cases. Antibiotic and antifungal treatments can wreak havoc on our microflora through both short-term and long-term changes in the composition of the normal balanced microbiome. Antibiotics kill bacteria in our bodies and in the bodies of animals, but they can't distinguish between the good bacteria and the problematic bacteria. While we may eliminate a certain bacteria that is causing an acute condition, we simultaneously wipe out our necessary, beneficial microflora, setting our bodies off balance. My son's dysbiosis was likely caused by the antibiotics that I was taking just prior to his birth and through the first five days of his life. The antibiotics compromised the flora in the birth canal as well as shifted the microbial diversity in my colostrum and early breast milk. In addition, I passed on some of the antibiotic through my breast milk, giving my son his own dose of bacteria killers. Research is showing how crucial the mother's microbial balance is for the health of her newborn baby. It is her microflora that is passed on to her baby, which then initiates his flora—the very foundation for his long-term health. Antibiotics contribute to a dysbiotic flora in the mother, the effects of which are passed on to the infant during birth.[6]

Unfortunately, treating an infection is not the only way that antibiotics find their way into our system. We are also exposed to antibiotics from residues in water systems from flushed human waste and animal-waste runoff. Some critics even claim that antibiotics are transferred to us through the antibiotic-contaminated meat that we consume. This overexposure to antibiotics is having a significant negative impact on our microflora.

In the mid-1940s, ranchers realized that they could increase their profits by giving small doses of antibiotics to their animals, which would make most animals gain as much as 3 percent more weight. In an industry where profits are measured in pennies per animal, the gains achieved through routine antibiotic use were innovative and revolutionary. Today antibiotics are still routinely fed to livestock, poultry, and fish on industrial farms to promote faster growth as well as to pre-medicate for common illnesses that arise from the unsanitary conditions common in this type of production. Approximately 80 percent of all antibiotics used in the United States are fed to farm animals. This means that in the United States only 20 percent of antibiotics, which were originally developed to protect human health, are actually used to treat infections in people.[7] The problem with all of the antibiotics that we are using in animals is that they contribute to antibiotic-resistant strains of bacteria. Antibiotic-resistant bacteria are very hard to treat and contribute to infectious disease deaths in our country.

3. Increased Incidence of C-Sections

The moment of birth is significant to a newborn in many ways, many of which are quite obvious to parents. One less glamorous, and much less known, important occurrence at birth is the colonization of the baby's gut flora. While in the uterus the entire baby is sterile—inside and out. Upon leaving the womb and entering the world the infant needs to start building his microflora that will keep him healthy. The intestinal flora gets established through the natural birthing process. When a baby is delivered naturally she gets colonized by collecting bacteria and other microbes from the vaginal canal. When a baby is delivered via C-section, she is colonized by human skin when held as well as opportunistic bacteria in the operating room. The microorganisms that colonize a baby through the birth canal are very different than the microorganisms from skin; the latter being less balanced and suited to the needs of our immune system and gastrointestinal health. One in three babies in America are born via C-section, leaving many newborns with a potentially compromised start to health.

4. Decline in Breastfeeding

Breastfed babies receive microbes from their mother's milk which nurtures early microbial colonization of their gut. This enhances the expression of genes involved in immunity. The end result is that breastfed babies show enhanced resistance to pathogens. Babies who are not breastfed do not receive the same colonization from formula as they would from breast milk. The gut health that we develop as infants significantly influences our gut health as adults and directly affects how well our bodies function.[8]

Building the Microbiome

We have more microbiome DNA than human DNA. These microbes are obviously a significant part of our bodies that help us function optimally. We all would benefit from placing attention on the health of our microbiome in order to optimize our health. Here are a few simple ways to shift your microbiome and keep your gut flora on track:

1. Limit Processed Foods and Eat More Real Foods

Yes, this again! Plant-heavy diets are especially helpful for improving your microbial diversity, so hit the produce aisle hard and frequently.

Why? Because plants give your microbes something to chew on, to break down, to digest and extract the nutrients from. You are literally feeding the good little critters what they love and need to survive. Vegetables, fruits, beans, and whole grains create a healthy, strong, and well-armed microbiome that has the ability to keep us healthy and kickin' for a long time. Pile on the plants and enjoy.

At the same time, it is imperative to drastically reduce refined grains, sugar, genetically modified ingredients, processed foods, and pasteurized foods. These foods feed harmful bacteria and don't give the good guys what they need to flourish.

2. Decline Antibiotic Use Unless Necessary

Strive to keep your microflora balanced by taking as few courses of antibiotics as possible. This will help minimize the destructive effect antibiotics have on our intestinal microbes. Antibiotics indiscriminately take out everything in their path, including the good gut flora our body needs to support long-term health. When your doctor or dentist prescribes antibiotics, politely but firmly ask if they're absolutely necessary. If the answer is yes, then insist on the shortest course possible, use probiotic supplementation (discussed below), and increase your intake of fermented food (discussed below) while on the antibiotics and for a period of time after the course is over. Taking antibiotics when I gave birth to my son was not an absolutely necessary course of treatment. I started the treatment to decrease symptoms and to heal my respiratory tract infection more quickly. Knowing what I know now about antibiotics and the impact on infant health, I would have declined the antibiotics and used other means to treat my symptoms and heal my body efficiently.

3. Probiotic Supplementation

If you have to take an antibiotic, most definitely take probiotics to balance the impact. It is advised to separate the time of day at which the antibiotic and the probiotic are taken to help maintain the diversity of your microflora. Not on antibiotics? Take probiotics anyway. Doing so will help keep your microbiome full of live, beneficial organisms which will help keep digestion, immunity, and overall health on track.

Look for probiotics that deliver twenty to fifty billion live organisms per dose and contain a combination of different strains of Lactobacillus and Bifidobacteria.[9] Take probiotics as directed, once or twice a day, preferably with meals. I rely on the guidance of my naturopath to help me identify the best probiotic supplements for my family. Gravitate towards companies that have good reputations for quality products as there is some evidence that the quality of the probiotic can vary significantly. Also keep in mind that supplementation is exactly that, supplementation. It is no substitution for healthy eating.

4. Eat Fermented Foods

Consuming naturally fermented foods is one of the best ways to optimize your microbiome and digestive health. These fermented goodies like sauerkraut, kimchi, yogurt, kombucha, kefir, and pickled veggies encourage the growth of good bacteria. Add to that some pre-biotic foods, which are non-digestible short-chain fatty acids that help your good bacteria flourish. Pre-biotic foods include artichokes, garlic, beans, oats, onions, and asparagus.

Consuming one-quarter to one-half cup of fermented veggies with each meal is a good goal to eventually reach, but you may need to work up to it. Consider starting with just a teaspoon or two a few times a day and increase as tolerated. You can even begin by drinking a teaspoon of the brine from the fermented veggies, which is rich in the same beneficial microbes. If you regularly eat fermented foods your healthy gut bacteria will thrive.

It is important to know what fermented foods have adequate amounts of good bacteria because we can easily confuse products unknowingly. For example, I often hear people say they eat yogurt regularly in order to get probiotics into their diet. Conventional store bought yogurt is usually full of sugar and has very little probiotic properties. See the chart below for ways to ensure our food is fermented and helping us rebuild our microflora.

Probiotic Source	Considerations
Yogurt	You can buy yogurt at the store, but ensure that it contains "live cultures." Conventional store-bought yogurts often don't have the amount of cultures needed to be beneficial to flora and can be more like candy with all of the added sugar. You may be able to find plain yogurt with adequate "live cultures" in a health food store. Homemade plain yogurt is fairly easy to make. Many yogurts usually contain about two strains of probiotic—less than kefir.
Kefir	Kefir is a fermented milk drink made with kefir grains. It typically contains twelve to fourteen different strains of probiotics (significantly more than yogurt). Limit/avoid store bought kefirs that contain a lot of added sugar. The live cultures might be good for us, but the high sugar content can be counterproductive. You can purchase kefir with coconut milk if you are avoiding dairy.
Kombucha tea	Kombucha is a fermented tea. Raw kombucha tea can be made at home or bought in both health food and many conventional stores. Kombucha that does not claim to be "raw" in the ingredients may not be an effective source of live cultures. Pasteurization can kill the cultures that make kombucha beneficial.
Sauerkraut, pickles, kimchi, and other fermented veggies	Fermented pickles, sauerkraut, and other pickled foods made with salt water and left to ferment contain healthy live cultures. You can make your own at home or you can purchase fermented food at a health food store. If you purchase fermented food, ensure that it contains "live cultures." Many conventional store bought pickled veggies are made from vinegar and lactic acid and do not contain "live cultures," thus are not effective in building gut flora. Store bought pickles often contain corn syrup also—yuck!
Miso soup	Miso is a traditional Japanese seasoning made from fermented soybeans with salt and fungi. You add this paste to broth to make soup. You can buy miso paste in health food stores. If you use miso in soups, be aware that high heat will kill the bacteria.
Tempeh	Tempeh is fermented soybeans. You can make your own tempeh at home or buy it in a conventional or health food store.
Probiotic supplements	Not all probiotics are created equal. I rely on my naturopathic doctor for guidance regarding probiotic supplementation. Probiotics in your local grocers or drug store may not be effective. Find high quality brands that are trusted and have been proven effective. Rotation of probiotics is a good idea to introduce your gut to many different types of bacteria over time.

5. Bring The Great Outdoors In

One of the best and potentially most pleasurable ways to increase our microbial exposure is to simply open the windows and let the microbes flow! Welcome them into your home, your car, your office—the more, the merrier, and the better for our microbiome. Next, get outside and get your hands dirty. Do some gardening, plant some flowers, mow your lawn, or do any activity that will connect you and your immune system with the trillions of microbes in the soil. There are new studies looking at the impact of soil health on our health. Apparently, fruits and vegetables grown in soil with diverse microbes actually pass that variety on to us. Unfortunately, conventional growing practices deplete the microbial diversity of the soil, reducing our overall exposure to beneficial bugs. Loving on pets is another great way to be exposed to healthy bacteria.

6. Stay Away From Antibacterial Hand-Sanitizers

These days most of us spend the majority of our lives indoors, stuck in cars, homes, and offices, frequently dousing ourselves in antibacterial cleansers. Sure, we're "clean," but we're also severely limiting our exposure to a wide diversity of microbes, whose presence in our guts (and on our skin) have a protective, immune-boosting effect. In other words living in the germ-free bubble that so many of us find comfortable is actually making us less able to fend off illness and disease. This is the opposite of what all that cleanliness was supposed to do in the first place. To combat this health-compromising, sterile lifestyle and to strengthen our immune system, step away from the Purell and start exposing yourself, microbially that is. Using soap with antibacterial products will kill skin microflora, which we need to build our intestinal flora. These products also often contain a chemical called triclosan, which has been linked to hormonal problems in animals. Instead, wash with soap that is not antibacterial. According to the Centers for Disease Control and backed by a wealth of research, washing hands with ordinary soap and water sufficiently removes harmful germs. Work the soap into a lather, rub your hands together for at least twenty seconds (sing "Happy Birthday" twice) and rinse well. Don't forget to scrub under nails and up the wrist.[10]

Avoid being excessively concerned about germs. Raising kids in semi-sterile environments sabotages their immune systems. Kids who are raised with animals or dirty environments have been shown to have lower rates of asthma and most allergies. The percentage of germs that can hurt us is very tiny, especially when we have a strong microbiome and, therefore, a strong immune system. My naturopath says that it is not the germ that is the problem; it is the health of the terrain it is entering that sets us up for disease or resistance.

7. Developing A Healthy Gut Flora Begins At Birth

Childbirth and breastfeeding set the stage for what organisms are going to inhabit a baby's body. Therefore, if you're a mother-to-be, it's important that you optimize your own microflora as you will be passing it along to your child. During your baby's first few months, he relies on your breast milk to help inform his immune system about what's dangerous. This is the beginning of natural immunity. If you had a C-section or were unable to breastfeed, don't beat yourself up. Simply be aware that your child's gut flora may need a little extra attention to build it up for strong immunity. If you notice that your infant is fussy, has colic symptoms, or spits up often, then you might consider seeing a naturopath or medical doctor familiar with the microbiome for support in building a healthy gut flora. There are probiotics designed for infants. It can also be beneficial for breastfeeding mothers to remove certain foods that can be common intolerances, like dairy, corn, eggs, soy, and/or wheat for a period of time while the infant's gut is able to heal and build its own healthy microbiome.[11]

Inflammation in the Gut

It was briefly mentioned earlier that inflammation and intestinal flora have a two-way relationship; they impact each other directly. Let's explore the concept of inflammation a little deeper. Due to our lifestyle of poor eating and sleeping, high levels of stress, and microbial dysbiosis, we tend to have significant inflammation, both locally in our gastrointestinal (GI) systems as well as systemically throughout our bodies—often without even knowing it. If you have a well-functioning digestive system and intestinal flora, your overall health is probably better than the majority of the population due to lower levels of overall inflammation. But as our gut flora changes for the worse, inflammation ensues. On a local level harmful microbes cause the intestinal lining to get irritated and inflamed. When my son's intestinal yeast infection was at its worst, he was irritable, in pain, had diarrhea, and constantly drank water—day and night. It was as if his intestinal tract was on fire. This was the result of local inflammation from the yeast irritating his intestinal lining. We also get systemic inflammation when dysbiosis causes the stomach lining to become permeable, resulting in an immune attack against foods and toxins that make their way into places they shouldn't be. The process that contributes to systemic inflammation is explained in the section below. My son's systemic symptoms from dysbiosis were eczema, irritability, interrupted sleep, anger, sensitivity to touch, and black-out crying spells. Over time, if we do not recognize symptoms as cellular inflammation and address the root causes, our immunity becomes compromised, and more toxins, chemicals, bacteria, and even parasites further irritate the lining of the stomach—inflammation worsens and the spiral continues.

Food Allergies and Sensitivities

Food allergies and sensitivities (sometimes called food intolerances) are major contributors to inflammation. We are experiencing an outbreak in food sensitivities, and it's not just buzz. In addition, both environmental and food-borne allergies are on a rise across the board. Up until recently, problems with food were thought to only be caused by allergic reactions, manifesting as swollen lips and throat, extreme diarrhea, uncomfortable rashes, and breathing problems. We are now learning that our bodies can be "sensitive" to food in a less obvious manner that can nonetheless have both physiological and mental consequences. Let's tease out the difference between food allergies and food sensitivities.

Food allergies and food sensitivities trigger the immune system differently. A food allergy triggers a histamine response from the immune system. This response can translate into experiences of sniffles, a scratchy throat, itching, trouble breathing, swelling, hives, or in the worst case, an anaphylactic reaction. We all probably know someone who can have an allergic reaction to something (food or environment triggered). With an allergy, we have an initial exposure that sets up the immune reaction but doesn't cause severity of symptoms with the first contact. However, the reaction will then occur every time that food is consumed, and often each subsequent exposure causes a worse reaction than the previous.

Food sensitivities can be less obvious and more difficult to recognize because they can creep up on us over time, and the entire body can be affected, making it confusing to know how to pinpoint cause and effect. However, these are still immune responses—delayed immune responses. The definition can be as ambiguous as this one presented by Dr. Susan Blum, Functional MD and author of *The Immune System Recovery Plan.* She says, "You feel better when you don't eat it and you feel worse when you do." Food sensitivities can be difficult to identify because they can cause almost any symptom. Common gut related symptoms are gas, bloating, constipation, heartburn, and diarrhea. Other symptoms are feeling puffy or swollen, brain fog, fatigue, skin rashes, weight gain, acne, irritability, depression, headaches, arthritis, and muscle pain. When you consider the subtle nature of some of these symptoms, you can appreciate why many sensitivities often go undiscovered. In addition, for many of us the symptoms may not be significant enough for us to even recognize them as a serious long term problem. We often don't readily connect our symptoms with the problematic food because food sensitivities may take days, weeks, or months from the time of consumption to arise. For all of these reasons we continue to consume the same offending foods and the inflammation caused by the sensitivity becomes chronic. It is worth noting that the foods that cause sensitivities are usually not in and of themselves "bad," but rather many factors such as inflammation and unhealthy gut flora can create an environment that makes it more likely for our bodies to react to a particular food.

Even individuals well into their adult years are developing food sensitivities. Why is this? How do we develop them in the first place? Food sensitivities are directly linked to the health of the intestinal lining, which houses our intestinal flora and immune system and acts as a defense against foreign substances that we consume. Dr. Blum explains this process in terms that are easily understood by the layperson, and I recommend her work if you are interested in more detail. The basic concept of how food sensitivities develop is roughly as follows: Our balanced, healthy, and intact gut wall protects us from directly absorbing non-digested foods or substances into the bloodstream, keeping the food within the digestive system. Our acids, enzymes, and bacteria break down most substances that we consume into unrecognizable elements, which our body easily absorbs. They pass into the blood, and the body and the immune system ignore them. But as our gut flora become compromised (due to overuse of antibiotics, poor diet, pollutants, stress, infections, and other factors), they are not as capable of breaking down or "destroying" some of the substances. In addition, the imbalance in flora results in a weakened intestinal lining, often leading to "Leaky Gut Syndrome." As these substances then pass from the digestive tract to the rest of the body (through this weakened intestinal lining) they maintain an identity that our body sees as a foreign substance. Our immune system recognizes these substances as "not us" and attacks the cells. Then, as the health of our gut continues to deteriorate, and we continue to consume some of the hard-to-digest substances (note GMO foods and gluten proteins are particularly hard to digest), the cycle continues. This constant immune response results in chronic inflammation, showing up as the symptoms mentioned above. A weak intestinal lining is most often the result of imbalanced intestinal flora.

Traditional allergy testing such as the IgE blood test or skin-prick test can uncover many food allergies. Food sensitivities, on the other hand, can cause so many different kinds of inflammatory reactions that they are often hard to identify with a blood test. This complexity is why they are often dismissed in conventional medicine and can be more difficult to diagnose or identify. Many of the blood tests that claim to uncover food sensitivities are scrutinized for poor validity, so their accuracy may or may not be consistent or reliable. Nevertheless, our family has had positive results using some of these tests to at least identify good places to start when our kids were exhibiting symptoms that did not have other diagnosable causes. If you have the patience and persistence, the "elimination diet" may be the best way to identify sensitivities. It is a systematic plan to remove and then reintroduce foods in a particular manner in order to identify those foods that trigger unwanted symptoms. Remove suspect foods from your diet for at least three weeks. If you don't have a sense of which foods could be the irritant, start by removing the five most common culprits: gluten, corn, dairy, eggs, and soy. You can identify the culprit by watching for uncomfortable symptoms when you reintroduce each food (try introducing one food every four days, consuming that food two to three times per day). For many of us, removing these common irritants is a great place to start in trying to identify the cause of our symptom(s). Although it is likely the most reliable way to identify a food intolerance, we have at times felt overwhelmed trying to successfully implement the elimination diet with our young kids (hence the blood tests that we have done). There are also other food-sensitivity tests that naturopaths have been using for years with successful clinical results. Working with a health coach, naturopath, or medical doctor familiar with food sensitivities is a constructive way to develop a plan for identifying problematic foods and take steps towards healing the digestive system.

The good news about food sensitivities is that we can often heal our digestive tracts—by removing irritating foods, rebuilding a healthy microbiome, and strengthening the immune system—and then subsequently reintroduce the offending foods back into our diet. As our body gets stronger, it is more able to tolerate some of these foods again.[12]

Gut Inflammation Affects Your Skin and Nervous System

Inflammation in the gut can manifest as diarrhea, gas, bloating, acid reflux, constipation, and other digestive symptoms. However, it also frequently manifests as skin conditions such as acne, eczema, rashes, rosacea, and dermatitis, since intestinal permeability causes both local and systemic inflammation.[13] Systemic inflammation frequently shows up on the skin and can even lead to skin disease. A study conducted in the early 1900s demonstrated that patients with acne were more likely to show unhealthy bacterial strains isolated in their stools, indicating a bacterial imbalance in the intestines.[14] Increased intestinal permeability has been shown to be a significant issue with people who struggle with acne, reinforcing the concept that inflammation in the gut may contribute to uncontrolled skin issues. When I eat foods high in refined sugar or simple carbohydrates, I break out in acne. This shows me that my body responds to these foods with inflammation. At about two and half to three years old, my youngest son had moderate eczema covering his back, cheeks, and trailing down his legs. He was itchy and had a hard time sleeping at night. We identified sensitivities to eggs and nuts (foods that he absolutely loved). When we removed those foods his eczema disappeared completely within two weeks. The direct improvement from the food removal was astonishing to us.

In addition to skin-related symptoms, intestinal inflammation can manifest in the nervous system, affecting brain functioning and mood. It can affect memory and even contribute to Alzheimer's disease. The receptors in the nervous system are very similar to the receptors in the intestinal lining of the gut, and the two systems are constantly exchanging chemical and electrical messages. This connection is so strong that many consider the gut our "second brain." What affects the stomach will directly affect the brain and vice versa. One of the many neural symptoms that my son had from intestinal inflammation was hypersensitivity to touch. He didn't like his skin lightly touched or massaged like my other two children. His resistance to touch quickly resolved when the inflammation in his gut was controlled.

The bottom line is that if you struggle with skin conditions, unstable moods, or GI issues you might want to consider starting from the inside out. Eliminating certain foods and rebuilding your intestinal flora can help with inflammation considerably and resolve long-standing ailments. Do your own experiment and see what results you get. It can't hurt to test the theories, and you may end up avoiding the use of unnecessary prescription drugs and antibiotics that could potentially worsen the problem. I suggest you start by seeking out a health coach, naturopath, or medical doctor who is familiar with the microbiome to help you assess your risk for yeast, bacteria, or other harmful overgrowth as well as food allergies and/or sensitivities that could be contributing to intestinal inflammation.

Stress: The Microbiome Nemesis

Food is clearly a key ingredient in supporting a healthy intestinal tract, balancing microflora, and maintaining low levels of inflammation, but it is not the only factor. In Chapter 4, we talked about many of the effects of stress and cortisol dysregulation, including weight gain, sleep disturbance, fatigue, a reduction in life span, and more. As noted in that chapter, stress also wreaks havoc on our digestion, immune health, and intestinal microflora. Many experts emphasize that stress management is as important a factor in bacterial balance and immune health as food.[15] We can eat a clean and healthy diet that is optimal for intestinal health, but if we live with chronic stress we are most likely negating all the good we do with the food. According to scientists from Ohio State University, exposure to stress leads to changes in composition, diversity, and the number of gut microorganisms. Research in mice has found that an increase in stress results in increases in the number of harmful bacteria and in a reduction of microbial diversity. Experimental studies have shown that mental stress slows down movement in the small intestine which encourages overgrowth of harmful bacteria and compromises the intestinal lining.[16] It's hard to overemphasize the importance of good stress management in overall health.

Controlling stress and anxiety has been a challenge for me personally. I can't lie—I have a handful of life stressors. I often fall into the trap of convincing myself that stress is harmless as long as I can simply maintain my responsibilities in life and *keep it together.* The truth is that this mindset underestimates the power and impact of stress on the body. Stress continues to show up as a significant player in various aspects of our health, so let's do something about it. Relax, try to be grateful for the blessings we have, slow down, and BREATHE! The benefits are countless and priceless. If you feel you have made a lot of gains in your physical health through diet and feel stress is still a major obstacle to your health, it's worth your money and time to consult a therapist who specializes in cognitive behavioral therapy and stress management to continue your journey to whole health.

Since our gut microbes are the frontline of our immune system and responsible for keeping all of our systems in check, it is vitally important to take care of them. Everything from our daily moods, to our skin health, to decreasing inflammation, and our chances of developing debilitating diseases rests largely on the health and strength of our microbiome. If we take good care of our one hundred trillion little companions, they will return the favor!

☑ LIVE IT. MODEL IT. TEACH IT.

LIVE IT.

- ☐ Give your gut some attention. Identify ways that you already take care of your gut and think of ways that you can improve how you feed those critical critters in your microbiome.

- ☐ Experiment with fermented foods and consider taking a probiotic supplement.

- ☐ Cut out antibacterial hand-sanitizers and soaps. Look at animal products that you are consuming, and if your budget allows, buy meats and dairy products from organic sources that have had less or zero exposure to antibiotics than conventional meats.

- ☐ Recognize how the health of your gut impacts your skin health, GI functioning, brain functioning, etc. When you recognize the interrelation of your gut with overall health, you can make better decisions about how you support intestinal health.

- ☐ Listen closely to what your body tells you when you eat certain foods. If you feel bloated, fatigued, constipated, foggy minded, or have other symptoms, experiment with eliminating foods to see if you feel better. The top-five food sensitivities in our country are dairy, wheat, soy, corn, and eggs. Eliminating one or more of those foods is a great place to start.

MODEL IT.

- [ ] Show your children what it looks like to value the health of your GI system. When you put a lot of attention towards helping your gut and immune system thrive, your kids will see the importance it plays in health and wellness.

- [ ] Talk to your children about food sensitivities you might have. Discuss discomforts when they occur, and brainstorm what you might have eaten to contribute to the sensations.

TEACH IT.

- [ ] Inform your children about gut germs. My children and I talk about the bugs in our bellies regularly. When we eat fermented pickles or sauerkraut we talk about how awesome it is that the food is feeding our friendly critters. One of my son's early words was "probiotic." I can't remember how he butchered the pronunciation, but he would ask for probiotics routinely.

- [ ] Teach your children how to support good bacteria in their guts (increasing vegetables, decreasing sugar, eating fermented foods, taking probiotic supplements, limiting antibiotic use, avoiding antibacterial soaps and sanitizers, not being afraid to get dirty, and managing stress well).

- [ ] Teach the family how to internally scan how their bodies feel after eating, and help them make the connection between food and how we feel both physically and mentally. Familiarize them with the concept of food sensitivities.

- [ ] Openly talk about how our skin informs us about the health of our bellies. A couple of my kids have had skin issues. We brainstorm ideas about why our skin might not be looking or feeling healthy and ideas that we can try to take better care of it. My three-year-old recently had an eczema breakout and together we brainstormed foods that we might want to eliminate from his diet to see if it improved. Together we decided he would try taking out chocolate since he had an increase in that food around the holidays.

12

Immune-Suppressed Society

In many ways we are making staggering advances in medical science and technology, yet as a whole we seem to be getting unhealthier. I have mentioned the increases we are seeing in obesity, heart disease, and other chronic diseases. But we are not only suffering more from chronic disease. Each year adults in the United States can expect to catch a cold two to three times a year, while children average six to ten annually, according to Joel Fuhrman, family physician and best-selling author. He asserts that the U.S. death rate from infectious diseases has doubled since 1980 and notes that infectious disease rates are higher now than at any other time in the last century.[1] In addition to the rise of infections, we are seeing increases in cancer (which we will explore in the next chapter). These increases are directly related to the health of our immune systems, or rather the poor state of our compromised immune systems. We are an immune-suppressed society, and we are feeling the consequences.

One of the most significant assaults to our immune system is—you guessed it: the standard American diet.[2] A diet high in manufactured foods, refined sugar, and unhealthy fats, and low in nutritional value reduces immune health, making us more vulnerable to infections and cancer. When properly nourished, our bodies can fight foreign invaders and protect us, even against cancer. Eating real foods is one way to give our immune-system cells the nutrients they need to thrive and do their work. At the same time, nurturing our "primary foods" is just as essential for maintaining immune health.

Some of the most significant threats to our immune system come from our tendency to neglect our primary foods. The immune system is directly affected by the resulting chronic stress, loneliness, sedentary lifestyles, and inadequate sleep. As we focus on food and the immune system throughout this chapter, it is critical to remember the powerful role that primary foods play in maintaining immune health. Remember, our primary foods are healthy relationship, meaningful work, regular physical activity, adequate sleep, and connection to your spirit. Part Two of this book introduced the links between all four of these "primary foods" and the health of our immune system. We must recognize that primary foods are the foundation for stellar immune functioning. This point is critical because even if we follow a healthy diet but lack primary food balance, our bodies will not be able to take advantage of the nutrients available. Stress, for instance, is a significant cause of immune deficiency due to cortisol release. When we are in a stressed state, we are unable to optimize absorption of vitamins and minerals. My naturopath believes that the single best way that we can strengthen our immunity, and minimize our risk for acute and chronic illness and even cancer, is by managing stress and finding ways to support a relaxed body state. As proof of this concept, mindfulness meditation (which supports a relaxed body state) has been shown to increase immune functioning. Remember also that lack of exercise and loneliness reduces immune functioning. Taking care of your primary foods and adding a healthy, nutritious diet to the mix will help you and your family build a superior immune system. Appreciating these links helps us move towards a lifestyle that not only impacts the way we feel and function on a day-to-day basis but also increases our life expectancy and nurtures a healthier aging process.

Immune System Basics

Now, with your primary foods in balance, let's get a better sense of what the immune system actually does. Just a friendly heads up—this section has a lot of medical language and in depth explanation of how the immune system works. If you would like to go deep, keep reading—if you would rather not, feel free to skip to "Focus on Function, Not Calories" on the next page.

Our immune systems are made of specific cells. These cells defend our body from invaders of any kind, like harmful bacteria, yeast, parasites, viruses, as well as substances like toxins and certain foods. I like to think of the immune system as a surveillance system whose sole purpose is to figure out what "is us" or what "nurtures us" and what "is not us" or "does not nurture us." It ignores the "is us" substances and attacks the "not us" substances.

The immune system functions through two primary modes. The *innate immune system* is the first line of defense and the *adaptive immune system* (triggered by the innate immune system) consists of a proactive attack against threatening substances. The innate immune system is a physical barrier, like a moat, while the adaptive system is dynamic, like archers on the tower shooting the invader. The skin, mucus membranes, and intestinal lining of the innate system keep the outside world out of our inside world. For example, the intestinal lining prevents the food that we eat from seeping into our bloodstream before being properly digested.

The adaptive immune system turns on when a foreign substance is identified in the body. This is typically the process we think of when we think about "the immune system." The adaptive system requires some time to respond (anywhere from hours to days) and actually maintains a kind of memory. Its armory consists of T lymphocytes and B lymphocytes (antibody producing cells). B lymphocytes kill invaders with bullet-like mechanisms—essentially they shoot and kill. The bullets are immunoglobulins (known as IgG, IgE, IgA, and IgM). T lymphocytes on the other hand are cytotoxic killers. They do their destruction by bumping up against the invader and releasing inflammation molecules to kill it. They are hands-on killers. These inflammatory chemicals and proteins that are released kill the invaders, but can also be irritating to us. This inflammatory response serves its purpose but is intended to turn off when the threatening substance is eliminated. The problem arises when the response is not turned off, resulting in chronic inflammation. As we learned in Chapter 3, chronic inflammation can cause local and systemic symptoms.

In order for our immune system to function optimally we need to find the cause of any inflammation and turn it off or avoid it. Dr. Susan Blum uses the "rule of tacks" to address inflammation. She says if you are sitting on a tack the answer isn't to take aspirin for the pain, the answer is to find the tack and remove it. We don't want to mask the symptoms of inflammation to merely feel better, we want to find the cause and remove it. The three most common causes of inflammation that negatively impact the immune system are: poor diet, dysbiotic intestinal flora, and food sensitivities. All three of these cause inflammation and all are interconnected. Poor diet causes an imbalance in flora, which causes food sensitivities, both of which can cause us to crave unhealthy foods which perpetuate the cycle. Research has validated this interconnectedness, concluding in one case that "The intestinal microbiota helps in proper development of the host immune system which in turn regulates the homeostasis of the microbiota."

We discussed the importance of a balanced microflora and the cascade of events that lead to food sensitivities in the previous chapter. Identifying food sensitivities and eliminating those irritants are crucial steps in the process of healing the microbiome and our digestive system and thereby optimizing immune functioning. If we continue to consume foods that are causing constant T lymphocyte attacks, we encourage chronic inflammation which is the precursor to chronic illness and decreased quality of life and can eventually lead to premature death.[3]

Focus on Function, Not Calories

What about the current American diet brings on such an imbalance in our immune system? We now know that the typical American diet is made up of 60 percent processed foods and only 5 percent vegetables and fruits. It turns out that vegetables, fruits, and other plant-based foods provide the majority of the nutrients that we need to support our immune system, while processed, refined, and simple carbohydrate foods not only lack any of these critical nutrients but have actually been shown to break down the immune system and promote disease. As a society, we need to move away from counting calories as a way to lose weight and supposedly "eat healthy." This common approach can easily lead one to believe that highly processed foods that are low in calories are a healthy choice. We must move towards a viewpoint that nourishing our bodies with real foods—packed with vital nutrients and powerful antioxidants—is the best way to lose weight, maintain wellness, and optimally support our bodies. Real foods help cells work properly, and processed foods cause poor cellular functioning. Food is much more than calories, and all calories are not created equal. This is especially true when it comes to immune health because immune cells are particularly sensitive to dietary compounds. For example, the nutritional value of a one hundred calorie apple is very different than the nutritional value of a one hundred calorie bag of pretzels. The nutritional chemicals and molecules in the apple penetrate our cells and influence how they will behave. The pretzel, a simple carbohydrate, on the other hand quickly converts into sugar which then penetrates and feeds the cells, creating sick and malfunctioning cells. As we learn how our bodily systems work, we begin to see food and calories in terms of function. In Chapter 10, we reviewed the importance of reading food labels. This is a critical skill once we understand what nourishes and what hinders our immune system.

The good news is that exceptional nutrition has the ability to significantly increase the protective power of our immune system, making eating well one of the simplest and most influential ways to strengthen our immune functioning.[4] Cultivating a healthy immune system sets us up to fight everything from colds and flus to cancer, impacting us in both the short and long term. Although optimal nutrition cannot protect us from every infectious disease nor ward off all cancers, it can significantly decrease our risk of contracting many common and serious illnesses. Using an ever-present analogy from the world-view of my three little boys, we could say that Americans' current diet is clearly heavily weighted on the "bad guy" side of the scale. Let's take a closer look at some of the critical players on both sides of the battle.

The Bad Guys

A general rule of thumb is to limit our intake of "white foods." These foods are often refined, processed, or simple carbohydrates. They are typically high on the glycemic index, limited in their nutrient value, and absent of phytonutrients. I consider foods like sugar, macaroni and cheese, bread, tortillas, crackers, breakfast cereals, chips, pretzels, pasta, and pizza as "white foods." There is a saying, "The whiter the bread the sooner you're dead." Not to say that anything that is not white is in the clear, like Oreos or Jell-O. Obviously, we have to use our critical thinking skills, common sense, and label-reading abilities to help us investigate and identify the "bad guys." And, of course, there are exceptions—foods like cauliflower, garlic, mushrooms, and onions are white but clearly do not count as "bad guy" white foods, as they are real foods and full of immune boosting properties. The more nutrient-deficient, processed, and refined foods that we eat, the weaker our immune system becomes, making us more vulnerable to infections and cancer.

The Good Guys

Not surprisingly, real food is where we find the "good guys." Micronutrients, found in plant-based foods, are critical to helping cells work properly and supporting an adequate functioning immune system. Dr. Fuhrman, author and physician, suggests that we need over ten times as many micronutrients (vitamin, minerals, antioxidants, and phytonutrients) for maximum immune function than we are currently getting. To a certain extent, we all know that getting enough vitamins in our diet is important; however, we don't hear as much about antioxidants or phytonutrients. Let's consider the importance of each of these micronutrient categories.

Vitamins consist of thirteen different substances that we need for normal growth and development. We need an adequate amount of these vitamins each day in order to support normal functions of the body. A deficiency in any of the following vitamins can lead to poor health, and sometimes serious disease:

- Vitamin A
- Vitamin C
- Vitamin D
- Vitamin E
- Vitamin K
- B vitamins: B1 (thiamine), B2 (riboflavin), B3 (niacin), B5 (pantothenic acid), B6 (pyridoxine), B7 (biotin), B9 (folic acid), and B12 (cobalamins).

Vitamins A and D take center stage when it comes to immune system health. The sun is a great source of vitamin D. You can also get vitamin D by eating fatty fish (salmon, tuna) and egg yolks. Foods with vitamin A include carrots, sweet potatoes, leafy green vegetables, cantaloupe, and bell peppers.[5]

Minerals are natural compounds formed through geological processes. Minerals are needed in the body in small amounts for proper functioning. There are fourteen minerals that have been scientifically shown to be essential for the growth and production of bones, teeth, hair, blood, nerves, skin, vitamins, enzymes, and hormones. Minerals are essential for nerve transmission, blood circulation, fluid regulation, cellular integrity, energy production, and muscle contraction. For example, iron aids the body in the production of oxygen-carrying red blood cells and can be obtained from beets, apricots, and kale. Zinc, in particular, supports our immune health. It helps heal wounds and strengthen the body's resistance to cold viruses; it can be found in whole grains, beans, and seeds. Selenium is found in Brazil nuts, mushrooms, whole grains, and seeds. These three minerals are particularly crucial for immune functioning. Yet too much zinc and iron can lead to health problems, so we must be careful to integrate the appropriate balance in our diet (especially if using supplements).[6]

Antioxidants are significant nutrients that boost our immune system and ward off infection, illness, and cancer. Their most critical role in immune function is the neutralization of excessive "free radicals" before they can damage our body's healthy cells. Free radicals are atoms or groups of atoms that have an unpaired number of electrons, making them unstable. These unstable atoms undergo an oxidation process in which they react with other cells, leaving behind new free radicals. As free radicals spread they can react with important cells (like DNA) and cause significant damage to critical cells, destroy normal tissues, and increase the concentration of cellular toxins. This destruction will continue unless an antioxidant halts the process. Antioxidants can bind to free radicals and interrupt the cycle by reversing or limiting the damage. Antioxidants are, therefore, a critical component to containing this chain-reaction process. They are found in brightly colored foods, especially those that are purple, blue, red, orange, and yellow—beets, berries, tomatoes, oranges, and lemons, for example. They are also present in raw garlic, mushrooms, nuts, whole grains, fish, and dark chocolate. Examples of antioxidant substances are vitamins C and E, lutein, lycopene, beta-carotene, coenzyme Q10, flavonoids, and lipoic acid.[7]

Phytonutrients are found in plant-based foods that work in partnership with vitamins and minerals to promote optimal health and immune functioning. They are compounds that protect plants against harmful entities like bacteria and fungus. There are more than twenty-five thousand different types of phytonutrients found in plant foods (including some vitamins like vitamins A, C, E, K, and folate). In some cases phytonutrients produce antioxidant effects. They stimulate immune function by building detoxification enzymes, positively affecting hormones, and acting as anti-carcinogen, antibacterial, and anti-viral agents. Fruits and vegetables are the most concentrated sources of phytonutrients. Other plant foods like whole grains, legumes/beans, nuts, seeds, herbs, and spices also contain phytonutrients. Common examples of phytonutrients include carotenoids, ellagic acid, flavonoids, resveratrol, glucosinolates, and phytoestrogens.

Carotenoids create vibrant colors in fruits and vegetables, like yellow, orange, and red. Carotenoids act as an antioxidant, tackling harmful free radicals that would otherwise damage tissue in the body. Some carotenoids are turned into vitamin A which helps your immune system work properly and is important for eye health. The following table highlights good sources of carotenoids.

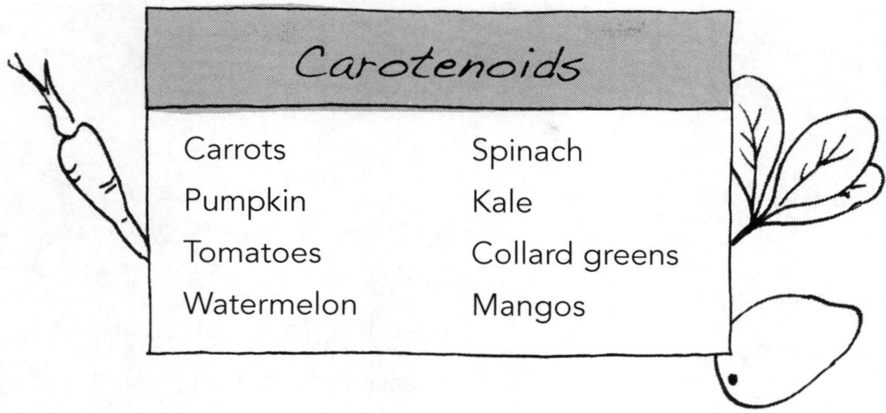

Carotenoids	
Carrots	Spinach
Pumpkin	Kale
Tomatoes	Collard greens
Watermelon	Mangos

Ellagic Acid is found in a number of berries and other plant foods. They may help prevent cancer by slowing the growth of cancer cells and helping your liver neutralize cancer-causing chemicals. The table below highlights good sources of ellagic acid.

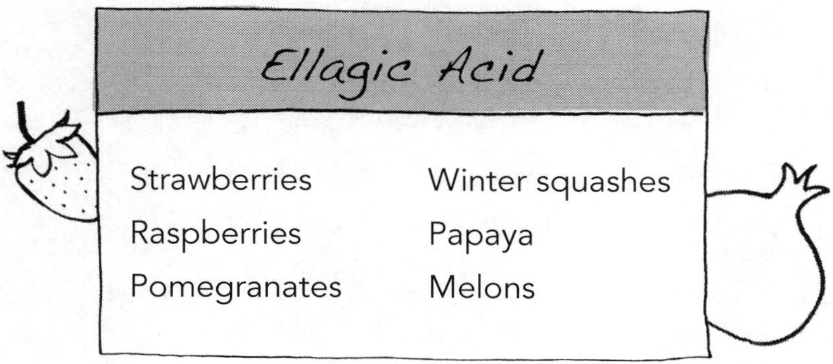

Ellagic Acid	
Strawberries	Winter squashes
Raspberries	Papaya
Pomegranates	Melons

Flavonoids encompass a large number of phytonutrients. Flavonoids are powerful antioxidants. Catechins can prevent certain cancers. Hesperidins can reduce inflammation in the body. Flavonols, like Quercetin, can reduce asthma, protect against certain types of cancers, and decrease risk of coronary heart disease. Resveratrol acts as an antioxidant and anti-inflammatory, and has been shown to decrease the risk of heart disease and cancer, and may help extend life. Glucosinolates, found in cruciferous vegetables, are powerful protectors against cancer. The list goes on. The table below highlights good sources of flavonoids.

Flavonoids	
Green tea (catechins)	Purple grape juice and wine (resveratrol)
Citrus fruits (hesperidins)	Cabbage (glucosinolates)
Apples (quercetin)	Kale (glucosinolates)
Berries (quercetin)	Brussels sprouts (glucosinolates)
Kale (quercetin)	Broccoli (glucosinolates)
Onions (quercetin)	Bok Choy (glucosinolates)

Phytoestrogens, like isoflavones and lignans, can block the effects of naturally produced estrogen, potentially decreasing the risk of endometrial cancer and osteoporosis. The below table highlights good sources of Phytoestrogens.

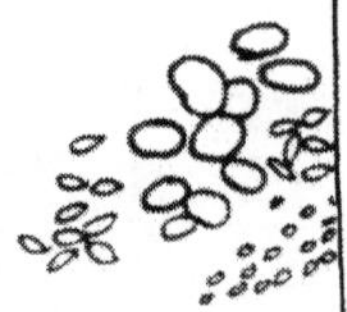

Phytoestrogens
Soy (isoflavones)
Flaxseed (lignans)
Sesame seeds (lignans)

It is important to consume vitamins, minerals, phytonutrients and antioxidants in their whole food forms and not just in synthetic form (a vitamin supplement, for example). It is easy to focus on the health benefits of a certain nutrient, but when isolated these compounds can at times offer limited benefit as they are most powerful when consumed in combination. Whole foods often have additional cofactors and enzymes (some understood and others still unknown) which enhance the absorption of the powerful nutrients.

Generally speaking it is best to get these micronutrients by eating the whole foods that contain them. Each of us has to find a strategy that works best for our family and is sustainable. In our house we strive to eat a good mix of real foods to get the nutrients we need, but we also do take a multi-vitamin on a regular basis to supplement these efforts. When my family is trying to ward off illnesses that we are exposed to, we combine strategies, increasing consumption of vegetables and berries, avoiding sugar and simple carbohydrates, and increasing supplementation (like Vitamin D, probiotics, black elderberry syrup, zinc, and herbal remedies). We also take antioxidant formulas throughout the winter months to help strengthen our immune system since we are at greatest risk for viral infections during those times. Similarly, your family can use this information to experiment with strategies that are practical for your situation and lifestyle preferences.[8]

Microbiome, Significant Yet Again

In addition to micronutrients like vitamins, minerals, antioxidants, and phytonutrients, we cannot forget the importance of the human microbiome when it comes to immune health. It is impossible to separate our immune system from our intestinal flora. Did you know that 60 to 70 percent of our immune system is housed in our gut?[9] A healthy balance in our microbiome directly improves the function of our innate immune system, the first line of immune defense which provides a physical barrier to invading bacteria, viruses, and fungi.

We are learning more and more about how the gut flora affects and informs our immune system. We understand that intestinal flora strengthens the physical defense of the gut wall. Our intestinal flora activates functions in the epithelial cells that line our gut and protect us from pathogens. If beneficial bacteria are absent, those epithelial cells aren't able to do their job, and the physical barrier to infection is compromised.[10] This is how the cascading effect of leaky gut syndrome, food sensitivities, and chronic inflammation takes off.[11] Gut flora also affects the pH of the intestinal environment, making the gut more acidic and hostile to the invading microbe—this pH is also critical for vitamin and mineral absorption. Our flora competes with potential pathogens for space and food. If healthy bacteria consume the available food there is nothing left to feed the harmful bacteria. In addition, our gut flora helps regulate inflammation, as we have discussed, allowing for appropriate immune system response, but not chronic overreactions. Our healthy gut flora also produce various antimicrobial substances. One species produces antibacterial substances that fight bacteria like E. coli and salmonella.[12] As these examples indicate, the role of beneficial flora in our body is essential for optimal immune system functioning.

A growing number of researchers are exploring the connection between intestinal flora and the immune system. One research team injected two groups of mice with various viral germs.[13] One group of mice had compromised intestinal flora, and the other group had normal intestinal flora. The immune response in the mice with the compromised intestinal flora was greatly reduced and caused the disease to manifest in a more severe form. When the mice with compromised intestinal flora were given supplementation to improve their intestinal flora, their immune response improved.

It is critical that we pay attention to the gut health of our children to ensure proper exposure to beneficial bacteria. The best path to achieve optimal immune response is through early establishment of a healthy population of gut flora which is, ideally, first established through the natural birthing process. After birth we can support the growth and maintenance of beneficial bacteria by limiting sugar and processed foods and by increasing our children's intake of vegetables, especially leafy greens, and fermented foods. Probiotic supplements may also help. Our family increases our probiotic consumption when we have been exposed to a virus or know that a particular cold or flu is making its way through our community. See Chapter 11 for more specifics on how to cultivate a healthy, balanced intestinal population of microflora.

Our body is a miraculous self-healing and self-repairing organism that instinctually resists disease. A healthy immune system is resistant to foreign invaders and designed to destroy cells in the body before they become fully cancerous.[14] We now understand how the standard American diet causes incompetent immune functioning. The nutritional status of our bodies is critical in preventing viral and bacterial infections from taking hold, but it is also crucial in the role of preventing cancer. In the next chapter we will dissect the importance of real food in the war on cancer.

☑ LIVE IT. MODEL IT. TEACH IT.

LIVE IT.

☐ Build your immune system by increasing vegetables and fruits and decreasing sugar and processed foods in your diet.

☐ Notice whether you get sick more when you eat highly processed and refined foods. When you do get sick, reflect on your diet—and stress levels—over the previous weeks.

☐ During times of stress, work to focus on healthy eating since your immune system is already compromised. Don't ignore stress and be proactive with stress management.

MODEL IT.

☐ You will likely get sick less if you are proactive in your health. Others may notice that you are strong, healthy, and infrequently sick. It is inevitable that we all get sick at some point. In fact adults with strong immune systems will have one to two illness per year, and a child with a strong immune system will likely get sick three to four times per year. Increasing real foods, especially fruits and vegetables, will likely decrease the frequency of getting sick as well as the intensity and length of time that you are down when you do get sick.

TEACH IT.

☐ Help your family make the connection between immune functioning and food by teaching them how vital nutrients from vegetables and fruits protect us from illness.

- [ ] Teach your family how sugars and processed foods can weaken the immune system and make us more vulnerable to illness, especially during flu and cold season.

- [ ] Teach your kids that during times of high activity and stress their body may not actually be in need of sugary and processed foods but instead might be craving some healthy food and good rest to function optimally.

13

The Cancer Connection

I left nursing school with the understanding that cancer was treated with chemotherapy and radiation; that it was caused primarily by genetics; and that once you "caught it" you needed the medical system to intervene with aggressive treatments. Cancer carried with it a sense of desperation, helplessness, and extreme measures. This perspective followed me through much of my hospice work, where although I saw primary foods help improve the health of cancer patients, I also saw people ultimately succumb to its inevitable end.

Then one day I met an individual at a social event who mentioned that he was "managing" his colon cancer with diet and lifestyle changes. Although skeptical, I was also intrigued, and I began to ask questions. He informed me that instead of using medications to "fight" cancer, he was avoiding everything that he knew "fed" his cancer, while at the same time nurturing those things that helped his body "protect" him from the cancer. I sat still for a moment, letting the linguistic mind shift settle in. At first his stance struck me as irresponsible or perhaps reckless. My training inhibited openness to this new perspective. But he shared how he completely avoided sugars and almost all refined carbohydrates. He made sure he got a measured daily dose of sunshine, and he regularly visited saunas in order to raise his body temperature. He ate a ton of vegetables. As he spoke, it felt like my mind was being blown open. It was one of those rare experiences where you are flabbergasted by what you are hearing and don't know what to do with the new information, or with the person sharing it. This was such a different view than I had ever experienced. Then he told me that since implementing these changes he felt the best he had ever felt in his entire life. Here was a man with colon cancer telling me that he felt great.

I left the gathering fascinated, and I soon began to ask experts and naturopaths what they thought, and to read everything I could find on the topic. I was shocked as I dove into this new worldview on cancer. My own naturopath validated the impact that food has on cancer management. I learned of many people who had cured themselves of cancer with this approach. I learned that there is a strong connection between food and our ability to prevent and fight cancer. Now, I am certainly no expert on cancer and I deeply appreciate the complexities of both its causation and its treatment. But this new information has intrigued me enough to drive many of my own eating decisions, like limiting sugars and eating more vegetables. This new understanding of cancer impacts both what I eat and what I don't eat.

Cancer rates have been steadily increasing since 1930. The probability of any one of us developing invasive cancer in our lifetime is currently 44 percent for men and 37 percent for women.[1] That means roughly one in every two men and one in every three women will get cancer in their lifetime in the U.S. When cancer does hit us, most of us believe that we have become victims to cancer in this "wait and see" game of roulette. Despite popular belief, and what I believed for most of my nursing career, less than five percent of cancer is solely caused by genetics.[2] It turns out that the cause of most cancers is lifestyle factors, such as tobacco use, dietary and exercise habits, environmental toxins, and infectious agents. I have already shared that many of our lifestyle habits contribute to inflammation, and that inflammation turns out to be a major contributing factor for cancer. These new insights have shown me that we have much more control over our risk of cancer than I previously thought.

I am part of a generation that has been raised on processed and manufactured food, fast food, and junk food almost from birth. But these eating habits, along with other lifestyle factors, have been shown to contribute to changes in cellular DNA which can ultimately lead to cancer.[3] Because of our long-standing poor eating habits, most of us are faced with the challenge of not only avoiding further cancer-causing exposures, but also of repairing the damage that has already occurred. The good news is that in most cases we *are* able to prevent further damage and even reverse the effect of already damaged cells, with modifications to our diet. Extensive research has established the connection between food and cancer. In this chapter, I will share some of the basic findings. I also hope to inspire you to further investigate this connection on your own, especially if you may be at high risk for cancer or already have a diagnosis. Certainly I am not suggesting that these changes will prevent or cure cancer for everyone. But just as my eyes were opened by the experiences of others, I feel inspired to share some of these insights with the hope that others will feel empowered in the prevention and treatment of cancer. Likewise, making the shift to viewing cancer as something that we *do* have some control over has been empowering to me, and I hope it can be for you as well.

In Chapter 3, we reviewed the idea that inflammation affects every aspect of our health and contributes to many chronic illnesses and causes of death, including cancer. Epidemiological studies have shown that chronic inflammation predisposes us to cancer. The longer the inflammation persists, the higher the risk of cancer. An internal environment of chronic inflammation causes cell mutation and proliferation, contributing to uncontrolled growth of cancer cells and metastasis (spreading of cancer within the body). Inflammation is also "angiogenic," meaning it enhances a tumor's ability to recruit blood supply.[4] The link between chronic inflammation and cancer is interestingly not a new discovery. In 1863, the origin of cancer was hypothesized to be at the site of inflammation. Tumors have been said to behave like a wound that fails to heal. If you remember from Chapter 1, wounds activate the inflammatory response in order for healing to occur, but when the inflammatory response becomes chronic it causes long term damage to cells. Therefore, tumors can be largely the product of chronic inflammation, basically a wound that has never healed.[5] It's not enough to kill the tumors (cancer cells) that are caused in this way; the chronic inflammation needs to be stopped at its root cause.

My acquaintance who had colon cancer made me realize that our attitude about cancer is greatly informed by the way we talk about the disease, even more so than by its actual causes. In every case I can remember of a friend, acquaintance, or patient with cancer, I have always been told that the person "got cancer." This linguistic slant implies something very significant about cause and effect. This way of speaking about cancer reinforces in our minds that it is something that happens to us, something that we do not have control over. Although it may be true that we cannot control some of the factors that contribute to cancer, it makes me wonder if our language could on some level be creating a self-fulfilling prophecy.

Contrary to my previously held belief, did you know that we don't "get cancer?" To begin with, I have learned that every one of us has cancer cells in our body at any given moment. This was another mind-opening insight for me. We have approximately fifty trillion cells that are continuously dividing in our body to keep us healthy. If one of those cells "mutates," it forms a potentially cancerous cell. A healthy immune system will immediately destroy most of these mutated cells before they can replicate and become dangerous. A compromised immune system, on the other hand, among other factors, may not be able to handle these mutated cells, thus allowing them to replicate and grow, ultimately leading to detectable cancer. In addition, a healthy immune system can also prevent blood vessels from growing into and feeding cancerous cells, thus cutting off their growth potential.[6] Therefore, nurturing our immune system and our body's ability to defend against mutated cells, free radicals, and blood supply to cancerous cells enables us to better resist and fight cancer.

This information led me to ask, if our bodies are able to fight cancer then how do these microscopic cancer cells turn into harmful and even deadly forms of cancer? Learning about the mechanisms that result in cell damage, the first stage of cancer development, has helped me understand how the process evolves. When our body provides an environment where free radical growth can thrive, we become more susceptible to cancer replication. Science has shown us that there are many things that can lead to free radical damage and cancer growth, including overexposure to the sun, excessive alcohol consumption, pesticides, cigarette smoke, excess body fat, and processed foods. Experts assert that foods in particular have some very direct links to the overgrowth of damaged cells.[7] Therefore, although clearly not the only answer to cancer prevention, foods will be the primary focus of this chapter.

When we examine the pervasive ills of our standard American diet, we find that our diet and lifestyle habits contribute to just such an environment where our immune system is not able to ward off these cancer cells. Processed foods in particular introduce substances that trigger cancer growth mechanisms, causing cellular mutations that subsequently replicate, divide, and spread. When not stopped by our suppressed immune system, they eventually turn into full-blown cancer.[8] The good news is that we can support our body's ability to defend itself against cancer by focusing on foods that have been shown to support our immune system and resist the cancer propagation process.

In the previous chapter, we reviewed the impact of diet on the immune system in general. In the context of cancer we have seen that a healthy immune system, in addition to protecting us against infections, also has the ability to recognize when our own human cells mutate (the beginnings of cancer development) and quickly remove them. Thus, a healthy immune system is our first line of defense against cancer.[9] Due to this connection there is a lot of overlap between the foods that support a healthy immune system and foods that fight cancer, but the information in this chapter is specifically oriented towards the foods that support cancer-fighting mechanisms. We have already seen that food can be a powerful medicine. But did you ever imagine that foods could potentially be one of our best lines of defense against even our scariest enemy—cancer?

It was learning about the food-cancer connection that really convinced me to increase my intake of vegetables. The immune system's protective mechanism that works to prevent cellular damage to our DNA is only active when we eat vegetables (especially cruciferous and green leafy vegetables) on a regular basis. If we are not eating green vegetables, our natural cancer-fighting machine is not activated. The human immune system evolved with a dependency on green vegetables for normal functioning. We have strayed from that evolutionary eating habit as our societies learned how to manufacture and produce food, unknowingly neglecting this essential defense system. A diet comprised of only five percent vegetables clearly does not provide enough support to maintain adequate protective power.[10]

Remember how important antioxidants from vegetables, fruits, grains, and nuts are in building a strong immune system? They are also particularly powerful weapons against cancer. It is inevitable that all of us will be exposed to some level of toxins that cause free radical damage to our cellular DNA in our daily lives (pollutants, poor eating habits, toxins, etc.). Antioxidants that occur naturally in our body as well as those obtained from antioxidant rich foods are designed to prevent and repair this damage. In one study, people who ate a poor diet and smoked cigarettes were shown, not surprisingly, to have a higher risk of cancer. But when one group of these individuals was given more vegetables and put on a healthier diet, their risk of cancer was reduced. Many other studies have shown that populations who eat a much higher intake of vegetables have a lower risk of cancer.[11] Free radical prevention and repair via antioxidants is the first mechanism that makes plant-based foods one of our greatest, and most easily accessible, resources in the fight against cancer. (See chapter 12 for a reminder of the type and benefits of some common antioxidants and phytonutrients.)

In addition to the antioxidants that repair free radical damage, vegetables and fruits also contain anti-angiogenic substances that stop blood vessels from growing into and feeding cancer cells.[12] Thus, eating vegetables, especially leafy greens which are particularly high in anti-angiogenic substances, actually slows or stops cancer growth. The following are anti-angiogenic foods recommended in Joel Fuhrman's book *Super Immunity:*

Anti-Angiogenic Foods

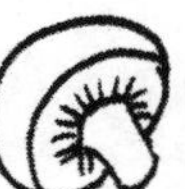

Allium vegetables (onion family)	Green tea
Berries (all types)	Mushrooms
Black rice	Omega-3 fats
Cinnamon	Peppers
Citrus fruit	Pomegranate
Cruciferous vegetables	Quince
Flax seed	Resveratrol (from grapes & red wine)
Garlic (raw)	Soybeans
Ginger	Spinach
Grapes	Tomatoes
Green leafy vegetables	Turmeric

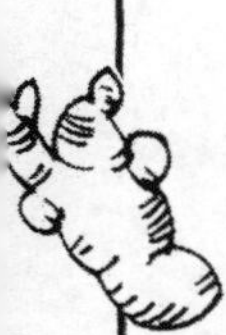

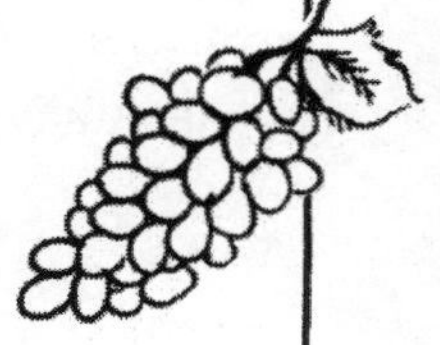

On the other side of the equation are foods and substances that promote angiogenesis, or encourage blood vessel growth into cancerous cells. Angiogenesis is activated by insulin, steroids, refined sugar, and processed foods.[13] Shifting our diet from one high in processed foods to one including more vegetables and fruits actually has the double effect of promoting anti-angiogenesis while cutting off the supply chain to angiogenesis. Now I understand what my colon cancer acquaintance meant by not "feeding" his cancer.

Green cruciferous vegetables, like broccoli, cabbage, kale, and bok choy, have a powerful ability to reduce cellular damage. Research has shown that there can be a 60 percent reduction in the risk of cancer when eating a diet full of cruciferous vegetables. In addition, eating large quantities of Chinese cabbage, kale, bok choy, and turnips has been shown to have a strong protective effect against breast cancer in women with the GSTP1 gene (a rare but strong genetic predisposition for breast cancer). Eating these vegetables suppresses the GSTP1 gene.[14]

Although green cruciferous vegetables can be a critical tool in cancer prevention, special note must be made about the body's ability to absorb their beneficial substances. When we eat broccoli, bok choy, or kale, we must chew thoroughly to break up the cell walls in order to expose the myrosinase enzyme (an enzyme necessary to form cancer-preventative compounds) to the glucosinolate (bitter, sulfur-containing glycoside that when hydrolyzed forms anti-carcinogenic compounds).[15] It is in the release of these two substances that the anti-cancer elements are formed. When eaten without thorough chewing, the essential anti-cancer compounds are not formed, and we lose the cancer fighting benefit of the vegetables. Blending vegetables in a high-speed blender—for green smoothies, like our family's "ninja juice"—is said to release the anti-cancer elements similarly to chewing.

It's hard to overemphasize the crucial role vegetables play in enhancing our natural defense system against cancer. The bottom line is to eat more vegetables, eat a wide variety of vegetables, and of course—chew them well!

Mushrooms can be another integral tool for enabling our immune system to fight cancer. Although lacking the micronutrients of vegetables and fruits, mushrooms have their own way of helping us prevent cancer. White, cremini, portobello, oyster, maitake, and reishi mushrooms have all been shown to have anti-cancer effects by preventing DNA damage, decreasing inflammation, slowing cancer cell or tumor growth, and preventing angiogenesis. Mushrooms support immune functioning by enhancing killer T lymphocytes which attack and remove infected or damaged cells. Essentially, mutated and damaged cells are more easily recognized as harmful by the immune system's T lymphocytes and are attacked before they turn into full blown cancer. Studies have shown that eating mushrooms every day reduces women's risk of breast cancer by 64 percent. And women in the study were eating only ten grams of mushrooms per day—about one button mushroom! Another study showed that mushroom extract was shown to halve the growth of breast cancer cells. That same study showed that combining a daily consumption of mushrooms and green tea reduced breast cancer risk by 89 percent.[16] Every woman in America needs to be aware of this powerful connection. Eating a mix of fresh mushrooms provides the best results, but even simple white button mushrooms and dried mushrooms initiate effective anti-cancer mechanisms.

According to Fuhrman, our cellular DNA is at greatest risk of damage between the ages of one and ten when we experience rapid development and cellular replication. Therefore, childhood diets play a major role in what will become our health as adults, and in part establish our risk level for cancer. This information is a significant motivator for me as I feed my children and their developing bodies. I am essentially setting their bodies up for health and longevity; what they eat now really matters for later. As for those of us adults who have spent years eating unhealthy, processed foods, there is also hope. We can make changes now that can heal much of the damaged tissue and DNA that has taken place since we were younger.[6] Reversing damage caused by years of nutritional abuse requires a concerted effort to fuel our body with high doses of potent foods that help us heal our damaged DNA and prevent cancer. Fuhrman outlines an accessible starting point for all of us, suggesting that we can reduce our risk of cancer by concentrating our dietary intake on his GBOMBS acronym.

Green Vegetables
Berries
Onions
Mushrooms
Beans
Seeds[17]

The ultimate fight against cancer consists of the following three interventions:

1. *Remember the anti-cancer foods contained in the GBOMBS acronym and consume as many of those cancer fighting foods as possible.*
2. *Reduce or eliminate as many processed, highly refined, highly sugared foods as possible.*
3. *Re-evaluate habits and lifestyle factors that contribute to inflammation in our body, and focus on practical solutions to begin reducing or managing those factors.*

It makes sense that any time we consume unnatural and noxious substances our body will have a negative reaction. The challenge lies in the fact that this reaction is usually not something that we immediately feel or notice. Therein lies the power of understanding how a compromised immune system can potentially lead to illness or cancer over time. Many of us have lived a great part of our lives underestimating the significance of the specific foods that we eat (or don't eat!). Unfortunately, it sometimes takes the development of a significant illness to push us to learn about these factors. Or, if we are lucky enough, we run into someone at a social gathering that plants some seeds that may eventually turn out to be lifesaving. That garden that your grandparents maintained with so much care represents the wisdom of evolution and tradition. It's time that we return to their example.

☑ LIVE IT. MODEL IT. TEACH IT.

LIVE IT.

- ☐ Be aware of the powerful relationship between food and the development of cancer.

- [ ] Be inspired to increase your consumption of anti-cancer *GBOMBS* foods in your cooking, snacks, and smoothies. Every day at our house starts with a green smoothie that is packed full of a variety of greens. In addition, my husband has been putting mushrooms in our smoothies, and we can hardly taste them. We sauté mushrooms in the mornings and try to add mushrooms to any dish that we can. We also try to have green vegetables with every meal.

MODEL IT.

- [ ] Eat well and reduce your odds of developing many cancers. Your family will learn a lot from your choices and behaviors surrounding food's ability to heal and protect us from cancer.

TEACH IT.

- [ ] Teach your family about *GBOMBS* and inform them about the way green vegetables activate important systems in our body to keep us strong and healthy.

- [ ] Talk to your family about the connection between food and cancer. Our bodies are strong machines that are meant to fight many of the diseases to which we have historically thought we were victims. We have the ability to prevent or reduce the severity of cancers through the food that we eat.

14

Moods and Foods

Like many others, I am no stranger to low moods. I have recently been exploring the connection between my diet and my moods and have been fascinated and inspired by what I've learned. Did you know that what we eat directly affects our mood? Perhaps you have noticed this connection firsthand. Depression is on the rise in the United States. According to the Centers for Disease Control, one in ten Americans report that they are currently depressed. Understanding the connection between food and our mental and emotional stability is critical because the current trend is to look to pharmaceuticals to solve our depressive—and other mental health—symptoms. These drugs can have side effects that threaten our health on many levels. The use of antidepressants has increased by 400 percent over the past few decades.[1] Many people diagnosed with depression are told that the root problem is an imbalance in serotonin—the "happy hormone"—in the brain, and some of the medications do effectively manage this problem. But this theory regarding low serotonin levels as the main cause of depression has lately come under scrutiny. There is a growing body of evidence showing gastrointestinal involvement as a major factor in a variety of neurological diseases, including depression and anxiety.[2] As I mentioned earlier, cutting-edge research is discovering the integral connection between the intestinal system and the brain, to the point that some now refer to the gut as our "second brain." Scientists have discovered that 95 percent of the body's serotonin lives in our intestinal tract.[3] In a very real sense we have two "brains" that both determine our mental state and mood. When we take care of our intestinal health, our brain and nervous system reap the benefits. Consequently, we are less moody, irritable, anxious, and depressed.

I have mentioned the food-related health issues that we had with our middle son. In addition to abnormal stools, he also experienced a host of concerning mood-related symptoms. He seemed to have severe anxiety, anger, agitation, and fear that manifested as frequent screaming episodes and sleeping poorly at night, both of which seemed to be related to some unidentifiable agitation. He would even black out regularly from out-of-control crying spells that appeared to be the result of simply being overwhelmed with emotion. In our journey to understand our son's needs, we were typically told by physicians that he was "spirited" or "strong willed" and there was nothing we could do about it except discipline consistently. My motherly intuition always sensed that there was something more going on, that he was struggling on a physical level. As we pursued many professional opinions we found that our intuition was right. He wasn't just a "difficult personality," he was physically inflamed and miserable.

As I've said, he had been exposed to antibiotics that I was taking at the time of his birth and during his first few days of life, which we now believe were likely the initial cause of a yeast overgrowth in his intestinal tract. That yeast overgrowth caused inflammation in his GI tract that subsequently caused many food sensitivities, which created even more GI inflammation, and ultimately widespread discomfort. When we finally learned about the connection between GI health and emotions, we were hopeful that his moods would become more regulated and stable after some TLC went into healing his gut. We treated the yeast overgrowth and eliminated the foods to which he had developed sensitivities. Almost immediately, his stools drastically improved, and much to our excitement his moods quickly followed suit. He started crying less often and less intensely and began sleeping through the night more regularly. The link between GI health and moods couldn't have been more obvious to us after this experience. How could something so complicated be really so simple?

There are a handful of ways to support emotions and mental health through the food that we eat. Approaches that aim to decrease inflammation may be especially helpful because growing evidence suggests a link between chronic inflammation and mood instabilities. The following habits have been shown to support mental health:

1. Eating regularly
2. Limiting sugar and refined carbohydrates (including refined flours and pulverized grains)
3. Nourishing your intestinal flora
4. Identifying food sensitivities
5. Getting sufficient vitamin D
6. Taking omega-3 fatty acid supplementation
7. Balancing primary foods

1. Eating Regularly

Food is our fuel, so doesn't it make sense that if we skip a meal we will feel depleted, tired, and cranky? If we don't fill our car with gas, we run out of gas. If we fill our car with the wrong kind of gas or cheap gas, it doesn't run as well and may decrease the life of the car. When we go too long without eating, our blood sugars crash and we experience mood swings. Eating a solid breakfast, for example, has been shown to reduce our cravings later in the day and can even reduce the amount of trouble that kids get into at school. Of course, we know that not all food is created equal, so it's important to eat healthy food at regular intervals. I often find when my kids are moody, irritable, agitated, or tearful, it is due to hunger. When I feed them a meal, they become happy and content. I can relate with my kids. On busy days when I skimp on meals, I am more cranky, anxious, and irritable. I even crave sugars more on those days. It is as if my body is screaming at me to nourish it better. These examples clearly demonstrate to me the impact of hunger and low blood-sugar levels on mood.

2. Limiting Sugar and Refined Carbohydrates

Sugar Blues, written by William Duffy in the mid-80s, delves into the sugar-depression link in great detail. Duffy argues that sugar is a health-harming, addictive drug, and simply eliminating as much sugar as possible can have a profound impact on your mental health. He even advocates eliminating sugar from the diet of the mentally ill, stating it could be an effective treatment in and of itself for many people.[4] Currently, sugar's effects on mood is widely written and talked about. *Junk Foods and Junk Moods* by Lindsey Smith is a great resource connecting how the junk foods that we eat directly impact how we feel and think.

It has become increasingly clear that one reason sugar is so detrimental to our mental health is because sugar consumption triggers a cascade of chemical reactions in our body that promotes chronic inflammation. We know that sugar leads to excessive insulin release, which, in turn, causes our brains to secrete glutamate in levels that can cause agitation, depression, anger, anxiety, and panic attacks.[5] This chain reaction has even been linked to an increase in suicide risk.

Consuming high amounts of sugar (more than 25 mg/day) pushes our brain biochemistry, and our overall health, in the wrong direction. I experience this shamefully during holidays, when I can lose all control and eat whatever sweet treat finds its way in front of me. After many days of this uncontrolled behavior, I find myself irritable, anxious, and melancholic. My experiences have validated this connection between diet and mood. I encourage you to pay attention to how your moods shift after a day of eating well versus after days in which you eat high amounts of sugar. The dietary answer for balancing mood is to severely limit sugars, as well as refined and pulverized grains (which the body processes similarly to sugars). This intervention fights chronic inflammation, high insulin levels, and, as we'll see below, supports healthy gut bacteria.

3. Nourishing Your Intestinal Flora

The microbiome's involvement in mental health is fascinating. A number of studies have demonstrated that there is a close link between intestinal flora and the central nervous system. It turns out that a balanced microbiome has a direct effect on brain chemistry, transmitting mood- and behavior-regulating signals to your brain via the vagus nerve. For instance, recent research showed the probiotic Lactobacillus rhamnosus was found to have a marked effect on levels of GABA, an amino acid that acts as a neurotransmitter in the central nervous system (low GABA levels are associated with depression and anxiety). Lactobacillus rhamnosus has also been shown to lower the stress-induced hormone cortisol, resulting in reduced anxiety and depression.[6] As we discussed above, sugar and refined carbohydrates affect mood. If we consume a lot of processed, sweetened, and refined foods (and drinks) our gut bacteria are going to be compromised and so is our mental health! Sugar does this by serving as a fuel for pathogenic bacteria, yeast, and fungi that negatively inhibit the beneficial bacteria in our gut. This imbalance in the gut ultimately affects our mental health.

Refer back to Chapter 11 for detailed information on supporting your gastrointestinal microbiome and decreasing inflammation in the gut. Fermented foods, vegetables, and probiotic supplements are a great way to build "good" bacteria in the gut. Limiting the use of antibiotics is an important way to keep the gut intact and healthy. Remember, when absolutely unavoidable, balance antibiotic use with probiotic supplementation.

4. Identifying Food Sensitivities

Evidence continues to grow that food sensitivities contribute significantly to the health problems of many Americans, including irregular moods and feelings of anxiety and depression. The nervous system regulates mood and emotional reactivity, among other functions. Recall that undigested food particles and toxins can seep into the bloodstream through gaps in the intestinal wall ("leaky gut"). From the bloodstream these substances can penetrate the blood-brain barrier.[6] The blood-brain barrier is supposed to protect the brain from such foreign particles, but once these foreign substances cross the blood-brain barrier our nervous system becomes inflamed and overstimulated.[7] The result is that we can feel out of control, anxious, cranky, and/or sad. Psychological signs of food sensitivities include erratic mood changes and emotional reactivity, out of control behavior (extreme tantrums and passing out in the case of our son), anger, rage, inexplicable sadness, and anxiety. Severe and intractable depression and anxiety can also be signs of an underlying food sensitivity.[8] See Chapter 11 to learn more about the physiological manifestations of food sensitivities. Work with a health coach, naturopath, or medical doctor familiar with food sensitivities to help you assess potential food sensitivities in your family and develop a plan to heal your intestinal integrity, immune system, and microflora. When we heal our body in this way, by addressing the root cause of the problem, we are likely able to eventually reintroduce the problematic foods back into our diet.

5. Getting Sufficient Vitamin D

Many of us are not aware that vitamin D deficiency is associated with depression. One study found that people with the lowest levels of vitamin D were more depressed than those who had normal levels.[9] Research shows that the lower a person's level of vitamin D, the greater his or her risk for depression. The simplest way to keep your levels in the healthy range is by getting proper sun exposure. Taking a high-quality vitamin D3 supplement is also a reasonable option since sunscreen can prevent adequate vitamin D absorption. This is especially true in colder or rainy climates where it can be difficult to get enough vitamin D from the sun during parts of the year. If going the route of supplementation, it is a good idea to have our vitamin D levels tested to be clear on what our supplementation should be. The amount of vitamin D supplementation needed can depend on latitude. In the northern hemisphere many of us do not receive much Vitamin D from the sun for a portion of the year. The recommended daily allowance for vitamin D is 800 IU for adults, but some studies have shown that we need much higher doses than this (more like 2,000

IU per day). Consult your health care practitioner, though, as Vitamin D can be toxic when high doses are taken over time.[10] According to the National Institutes of Health, children from birth to five years old require 200 IU of vitamin D per day. Foods rich in vitamin D include eggs, milk, salmon, tuna, mackerel, and sardines. To get adequate vitamin D from sun exposure, a practical strategy is to spend ten to fifteen minutes per day outside before applying sunscreen.

6. Taking Omega-3 Fatty Acid Supplementation

In addition to regulating inflammatory processes and responses as previously discussed, omega-3 fatty acids have also been shown to positively influence outcomes in depressive disorders.[11] Research shows that low omega-3 levels are associated with depression, pessimism, and impulsivity.[12] New research states that an omega-3 fatty acid called elcosapentaenoic acid (EPA) is as effective for treating depression as traditional anti-depressants. One study found that two thirds of the depressed individuals who took a daily dose of EPA had a 50 percent reduction in feelings of sadness and pessimism, inability to work, sleeplessness, and low libido. All of the individuals in the study had previously tried Prozac, other SSRIs (a class of drugs commonly used for depression), and tricyclic antidepressant medications. About 20 percent of brain cell membranes are made of fatty acids, making omega-3 fatty acids a critical ingredient to keep brain signals moving smoothly.[13] We can get these essential omega-3 fatty acids in seafood, walnuts, leafy greens, flaxseed, and chia seed, among other foods. Worth noting is that countries with diets rich in fish have lower rates of depression, bipolar disorder, postpartum depression, and suicide.[14]

If you are currently struggling with depression or other emotional turmoil, taking at least 2,500 mg of a high-quality omega-3 fatty acid supplement per day is a simple and smart choice.[15] See Chapter 15 for Omega-3 dosing suggestions for children. If your child is struggling with depression or anxiety it is worth working with a health professional versed in omega-3 supplementation to better understand a therapeutic dose for your child. Omega-3 fatty acids are not likely the only solution in this scenario, but they have the potential to shift things in the right direction. Ensure you are getting a high quality product by checking the label for third party testing, environmental toxins including heavy metals, dioxins, and PCBs. Read the label for EPA and DHA content, not just a total quantity of omega-3. I've found Nordic Naturals to be one reliable brand. It is a good idea to research products or ask a health care practitioner who is informed on quality supplements in order to optimize supplementation.

7. Balancing Primary Foods

Those of us who are less physically active, more isolated, sleep deprived, and do little to manage our stress are much more likely to have mood instabilities. Every one of the primary food components can negatively affect mood. Although food and nutrition are a large part of our emotional health, remember that the picture is much bigger than food alone. Following a real food diet, getting regular exercise, managing our response to stress, being in connected relationships with ourselves and others, and getting adequate sleep all reduce unnecessary inflammation and positively affect our moods. Giving attention to these components is the most powerful strategy to protect both our physical and mental health. As always, we need to think of our whole health. Interestingly, many developing countries and traditional cultures tend to have lower incidence of depression than the U.S. This may be a reflection of how our busyness and ambition to "have it all" may ultimately be setting us up for mental health issues.

☑ LIVE IT. **MODEL IT.** TEACH IT.

LIVE IT.

- ☐ Take care of your emotions by taking care of your second "brain"—your gut. If you are feeling emotionally unstable your diet is a perfect place to start to stabilize your mood. Begin by reducing or eliminating sugar, identifying food sensitivities, and rebuilding a healthy microbiome.

☐ We are busy! But we still need to eat healthy foods regularly. This is essential for blood sugar stability and to fuel our body with foods that nurture us instead of harm us.

☐ Observe how sugar affects your moods and focus on nutritious foods to heal any unstable moods. Consider doing an elimination diet to identify any potential food sensitivities that may be causing systemic inflammation.

☐ Take care of your micro-flora and get enough vitamin D and omega-3 fatty acids. Consider taking probiotic, vitamin D3, and omega-3 supplementation to support your emotional and overall health.

☐ Reflect on which primary foods you might be neglecting that could be contributing to emotional imbalance.

MODEL IT.

☐ Show your family what it looks like to explore the connection between moods and foods by talking openly about how certain foods make you feel good and others bring you down or make you irritable. Use your diet to take control of any unstable moods that you experience. Your family will likely be inspired and grateful for your commitment to tending to your emotional health.

TEACH IT.

☐ Teach your family about their second brain. Inform them about the connection between their gut and their emotional health. If you have a family member who is anxious, fearful, depressed, or experiencing other emotional challenges, work with a trusted naturopath or medical doctor to identify the underlying cause and develop a treatment plan that includes diet and natural supplementation.

- [ ] Help your family understand the importance of eating healthy foods regularly. This is especially important for teenagers who often skip meals or replace meals with sugary, starchy foods that provide calories but often have negative side effects.

- [ ] Experiment with omega-3, vitamin D3, and probiotic supplementation with the whole family and share your knowledge about the benefits of these supplements on physical and emotional health.

15

Influencing Inflammation With Food

In Chapter 3, we discussed how inflammation is part of the body's immune response; without it, we can't heal. But when it's out of control and becomes chronic, it can damage the body. We gain weight, get sick, and age faster due to high levels of inflammation. Inflammation plays a major role in most chronic diseases and in conditions like asthma and allergies. All of the disorders you are familiar with that end in "itis," such as arthritis and colitis, are caused by inflammation. Our diet is an important part of keeping inflammation in check because the food that we eat either triggers or curbs inflammation in the body.[1]

Cellular inflammation often occurs below the threshold of perceivable pain, so it's easy to unknowingly cultivate long term damage by leaving the inflammation unchecked. Conversely, if we can proactively control this often imperceptible inflammation, we can significantly control our long term risk of disease. We have what is essentially a master genetic switch that turns on and turns off inflammation in our body. Foods have a direct impact on this switch. Some foods, like omega-6 fatty acids, turn on the switch and increase cellular inflammation. High levels of omega-6 fatty acids are found in corn, sunflower, soybean, canola, and safflower oils. Unfortunately these oils are also some of the cheapest calories on the market and consumed excessively by Americans both knowingly and unknowingly. Saturated fats, like those found in red meat (especially corn-fed), along with excess simple carbohydrate consumption, also turn on the inflammation switch.[2]

So what turns this powerful switch off—and decreases cellular inflammation? Two substances in particular stand out: omega-3 fatty acids and polyphenols. Omega-3 fatty acids are most commonly found in fish, fish oil, hemp seed, chia seed, walnuts, and flaxseed. Polyphenols are chemicals that give fruits and vegetables their vibrant colors and work in our bodies as powerful anti-inflammatory agents.[3]

Many of our most commonly used medications are aimed at treating symptoms of inflammation and not the underlying root causes. According to Barry Sears, medical doctor, biochemist, and founder of The Zone Diet, there are three stages of disease:

1. *Wellness*
2. *Cellular inflammation*
3. *Chronic disease.*

At some level we have a state of wellness and experience cellular inflammation within a normal balance. Through exposure to environmental factors, such as diet, stressors, etc., we begin to increase the inflammation in our body until it manifests as illness or chronic disease. Finding our way back from disease to wellness can, therefore, be quite simple. We reverse the path of this progression and focus on reducing our level of cellular inflammation. Wouldn't it be nice to develop a magic pill that does this for us with no harmful side effects? If I could, I'd become one of the wealthiest individuals in the country. I hate to be the bearer of bad news, but there is no such drug. But, what would happen if as a society we began to see food as medicine, if we began to look for our treatments in the grocery store and in our gardens instead of at the pharmacy counter? The truth is that we already have this magic drug at our fingertips.[4]

There are three main categories of macronutrients in food: protein, carbohydrates, and fats. The fact is, we need all of them and depending on their balance in our bodies, they play a collective role in either increasing or decreasing inflammation. For example, recall that refined carbohydrates increase insulin levels. Under normal, healthy functioning, insulin is an important hormone that brings sugar from the bloodstream into the muscles and organs. But in large amounts, insulin can result in nasty side-effects, increasing inflammation and storing excess food as fat. Cutting out all carbohydrates is not the solution. We need complex carbohydrates (whole grains and vegetables) for brain health and normal body functioning. A deficiency of carbohydrates causes the brain to send a signal that increases the release of the stress hormone cortisol—and we already know that too much cortisol can wreak havoc on our bodies. Nutrition is all about balance. The trick is to eat in a way that nurtures the correct balance of the three macronutrients.[5]

Unfortunately, the standard American diet is not balanced and consists largely of foods that turn on the inflammation switch. Foods that are highly processed and contain refined sugar are the most significant pro-inflammatory culprits. In addition Americans typically consume a lot of refined white carbs, which are also highly processed.[6] The following table highlights common pro-inflammatory foods that are helpful to limit in our diet .

Pro-Inflammatory Foods	Examples
Polyunsaturated fats (high in omega-6 fatty acids)	Vegetable, canola, safflower, sunflower, corn, cottonseed, and soybean oils.
Sugar (or other high glycemic foods)	Candy, bread, pasta, granola bars, soda, sports drinks, fruit juice, cookies, cake, ice cream, cereal, dried fruit, and flavored yogurt.
Highly processed foods	Any food in a pre-packaged box, bag, or container that has high amounts of salt, sugar, artificial ingredients, and harmful fats. Most items in the middle aisles of the grocery store.
Processed meats	Hot dogs, lunch meat, and sausages that contain nitrites, chemicals, and preservatives.
Processed potatoes	Potato chips

Foods cooked at high temperatures	Fried foods and chips
Wheat (especially refined flour)	Bread, pasta, crackers, muffins, cold cereals, baked goods, and many processed, packaged foods.
Trans fats	Margarine, vegetable shortenings, partially hydrogenated oils in many crackers, cookies, and snack foods.
Dairy	Milk and cheese (the more processed, the more inflammatory, but even raw milk leans towards the inflammatory side).

Yes, this is a depressing list to read. It seems that we are called to decrease consumption of some of the most culturally common foods in our diet. Our comfort and convenience foods are almost all on this list. Believe me, I know it seems overwhelming to think about, especially if this is your first introduction to these limitations. However, over time I have found that the amount of good, rich foods that we are able to substitute for this list is as vast and exciting as this list is depressing and overwhelming. I encourage you not to focus solely on what you cannot have, but rather focus on the long list of amazingly delicious foods that are healthy and advantageous. The good news is there are many food options that turn off the inflammatory response and help heal inflammation. Substituting the following colorful, anti-inflammatory foods will give us more energy and keep our body ticking for a lot longer. Add the following powerhouse foods to your plate to curb inflammation:

Anti-Inflammatory Foods	Examples and Rationale
Omega-3 fatty acids	Foods that are high in omega-3 fatty acids include fish like black cod, salmon, sardines, and tuna, flax seeds, hemp seeds, green leafy vegetables, chia seeds, pumpkin seeds, and walnuts. You can also take supplements like fish oil, flax oil, and hemp oil if you don't think you are getting enough of this critical fat in the food you eat.

Fruits	All fruits fight inflammation because they are low in fat and calories and high in antioxidants, especially berries. Papaya has a particular compound called papain which is a protein-digesting enzyme that helps reduce inflammation and improves digestion.[7] That said, eat fruit in moderation as large amounts of fruit can also cause high blood glucose levels and large bursts of insulin release. These side effects can be counter-productive to controlling inflammation.
Vegetables	Cruciferous vegetables (broccoli, kale, spinach, bok choy, Brussels sprouts, cabbage) are highly anti-inflammatory (and as we learned provide powerful protection against cancer).[8] Beets have high levels of antioxidants and have been shown to reduce inflammation as well as protect against cancer and heart disease.[9] Please note that most nightshade vegetables such as potatoes, eggplant, and peppers are not considered anti-inflammatory.
Green leafy vegetables	Kale, spinach, collard greens, all cabbages, beet greens, dandelion greens, turnip and mustard greens, lettuces, and Swiss chard are examples of green leafy vegetables. These leafy greens are packed full of minerals and vitamins that are anti-inflammatory and anti-oxidative, such as Vitamin E, which plays a key role in protecting the body from cytokines (pro-inflammatory molecule).[10] The amount of flavonoids and carotenoids in leafy greens is impressive when compared to other vegetables.
Tart cherries	Researchers say that tart cherries may have the highest anti-inflammatory content of any food.[11] Note that sweet cherries do not have the same effect.
Ginger	Ginger is particularly helpful to reduce inflammation in the gut.[21]
Nuts and seeds	Almonds are particularly anti-inflammatory because they are rich in fiber, calcium, and vitamin E. Walnuts have high amounts of omega-3s which make them a powerful anti-inflammatory. All nuts are packed with antioxidants, which help your body fight off and repair the damage caused by inflammation.[12]

Olive oil	The compound oleocanthal, which gives olive oil its taste, has been shown to have a similar effect as NSAID painkillers (like ibuprofen) in the body.[1] It has the ability to protect the heart and blood vessels from inflammation, which is a great protection against heart disease. Not all olive oils are created equal, however. Many lower quality olive oils have been found to be low in oleocanthal.[13] You can test whether your olive oil has oleocanthal by noting if it has a peppery after taste when sipping a small spoonful.[1] You won't taste the peppery aftertaste in a cheap and ineffective olive oil. At high temperatures olive oil oxidizes and contributes to free radical growth in the body, so be cautious and only cook with olive oil at very low temperatures.
Whole grains	A 2013 Harvard study found that not all products labeled "whole grain" are much healthier than their more refined counterparts.[16] Ensure that the ingredient list has whole grain as the first ingredient and no added sugar (these criteria therefore exclude most breads, with some sprouted grain breads being an exception). Eating the grain in the whole form (not pulverized into flour) is the most nutritious way to consume grains.
Avocados	Some call avocados the world's healthiest food. Recent research shows that absorption of carotenoid antioxidants (lycopene and beta-carotene) increases significantly when a fresh avocado or avocado oil is added to a salad or other green. Avocados themselves also contain a spectacular array of carotenoids, which makes them a super-anti-inflammatory. The fat in avocados has gotten a bad rap over the years. In actuality, the fats in avocados actually keep inflammation under control.[14]
Tomatoes	Tomatoes are rich in lycopene, which has been shown to reduce inflammation.[15] Cooked tomatoes contain more lycopene than raw ones.
Garlic	Raw garlic has been shown to work similarly to NSAID pain medications (like ibuprofen), shutting down the pathways that lead to inflammation.[17] Garlic is known for its immune-boosting properties.
Onions	Like garlic, onions have strong immune-boosting properties. Onions contain quercetin and allicin which breaks down to produce free radical-fighting sulfenic acid.[18]

Grass-fed animal protein	Limiting the amount of animal protein we eat is a good idea. When you eat red meat make sure the cow was grass-fed. Conventional beef is typically finished with a high-caloric diet of corn, soy, and grains that are full of omega-6 fatty acids that increase inflammation. The meat of grass-fed beef on the other hand is leaner and rich in healthy omega-3 fatty acids and Vitamin E.[19]
Soy	The isoflavones in soy are said to make it anti-inflammatory.[20] However, note that heavily processed soy products are often full of additives and preservatives and are consequently pro-inflammatory. Be sure to find natural sources of soy or fermented soy products for the anti-inflammatory benefits. Good sources of soy are whole sprouted tofu, soy beans (edamame), soy nuts, tempeh, and miso (look for organic in all cases as most modern soy products come from genetically modified soy beans).
Dark chocolate in moderation	Dark chocolate is loaded with flavonoids, anti-oxidants that have been shown to reduce inflammation and protect the vascular system, heart, and brain. Choose chocolate that has a minimum cocoa content of 70 percent.[23] Avoid high sugar chocolate.
Turmeric	Turmeric is a common spice in Indian cooking. It is the spice that gives curry its yellow color. It contains a powerful compound called curcumin which helps reduce inflammation by turning off the switch.[22] My husband and I take a curcumin supplement daily from a reputable vitamin company. It is important that curcumin have black pepper extract included in the supplement to help absorption.
Kelp (kombu)	Kelp contains fucoidan, which is a compound that is anti-inflammatory, anti-tumor, and anti-oxidative.[24] Whenever possible get organic kelp that is harvested from unpolluted seas.
Red wine	Red wine contains a compound called resveratrol, which when ingested in moderation, has been found to have anti-inflammatory and anti-cancer properties.[25]
Green tea	The flavonoids in green tea are a potent and natural anti-inflammatory that have been shown to reduce the risk of heart disease and cancer.[26]

In addition to increasing our consumption of anti-inflammatory foods, it can be useful to take anti-inflammatory supplements to obtain necessary levels of omega-3 fatty acids. Our bodies thrive on an omega-6 to omega-3 ratio of 2:1. Our typical American diet is closer to a ratio of 10-25:1. The inflammation that results from this imbalance is damaging to our body. For almost all of us, achieving a proper balance requires decreasing our consumption of omega-6 fatty acids and increasing our consumption of omega-3 fatty acids. I am typically not a supplement pusher, but, as you can see, our culture is greatly deficit in omega-3 fatty acids. According to Sears, the average regular intake of these omega-3 fatty acids in America is about 125 mg per day, only 5 percent of what it was fifty years ago. In this case, supplementation is important because it is difficult to get enough omega-3 fats from diet alone. It would take six pounds of lobster per day, six pounds of tuna per day, or four ounces of salmon per day to reach the minimum daily recommendation of 2,500 mg of omega-3 fatty acids. There are well documented benefits of high dose omega-3 supplementation. High doses of fish oil positively affects heart disease, cancer, depression, attention deficit disorder, multiple sclerosis, brain trauma, chronic pain, osteoporosis, skin disorders, fertility, and weight loss, to name a few. This makes sense, right? Most (perhaps all) of these diseases and disorders are associated with inflammation. Although fish oil is the most common form of omega-3 supplement, there are good quality and effective algae-based vegetarian options that are now available. The more omega-3 fatty acids you can add to your diet the more you are able to put out the inflammation fires. Short chained omega-3 fatty acids found in flax seed, chia seed, hemp seeds, walnuts, and pumpkin seeds are often inefficiently converted to the long chain omega-3 fatty acids that provide the anti-inflammatory benefits, so it is wise to not solely rely on these foods for omega-3 fats (but that doesn't mean we should stop eating them!). It is important to get good quality omega-3 products. Some of the cheaper brands of fish oil have been shown to have environmental toxins, fillers, and/or use poor quality fish.

It's worth noting that we need to consume a therapeutic amount of omega-3 fatty acids to get a therapeutic effect. According to Sears, the following recommended doses of daily omega-3 fatty acids for adults depict how different types of people may require different levels of omega-3 fatty acid supplementation. Sears suggests that the body needs high levels to put out major inflammation fires. Although the recommendations in this chart should only be followed under the guidance of a health care practitioner, they are a powerful example of how different our needs can be depending on health status.[27]

Treatment Goal	Omega-3 Dose
Maintain wellness	2.5 g/day
Treat obesity, diabetes, and heart disease	5 g/day
Treat chronic pain (rheumatoid arthritis or cancer pain)	7 g/day
Treat neurological disease (Multiple Sclerosis, ADHD, Alzheimer's, depression)	Over 10 g/day

Please note that guidance from your health care practitioner is critical because high therapeutic doses can also thin our blood. If you are on other medications that affect the thickness of your blood or are about to have surgery, this can be a significant issue.

What about kid doses? The Food and Nutrition Board of the U.S. Institute of Medicine recommends the following omega-3 fatty acid doses for children:

- Infants zero to twelve months old: 500 mg/day
- Children one to three years old: 700 mg/day
- Children four to eight years old: 900 mg/day
- Children nine to thirteen years old: 1,000-1,200 mg/day
- Adolescents between fourteen and eighteen years old: 1,100-1,600 mg/day

All of my children take about 1,000 mg/day of omega-3 fatty acid supplements. I encourage you to understand your child's personal needs by working with a naturopath, health coach, or medical doctor versed in omega-3 supplementation to help you appropriately dose your child.

Food Sensitivities Ignite Inflammatory Fires

Food sensitivities and allergies are other factors that play a significant role in inflammation levels in the gut, wreaking havoc on the immune system and other digestion and neurological functions. As we discussed in Chapter 11, if we are allergic or sensitive to certain foods, those foods will act as an irritant and trigger inflammation. For instance, if you are allergic to dairy products, consuming cheese, milk or yogurt will cause gastrointestinal inflammation and will make you feel mildly to severely ill. Apart from local gastrointestinal distress, many people report systemic inflammation that can show up as anxiety or acne from sensitivities. Identifying sensitivities and removing problematic foods is important to address inflammation in the body.

☑ LIVE IT. **MODEL IT.** TEACH IT.

LIVE IT.

- ☐ Reflect on the foods you eat that may contribute to inflammation. Remember, the more our food is processed and refined, the more likely it is to cause inflammation and disease. Challenge yourself to decrease or even eliminate some of the most frequent or serious offenders.

- ☐ Review the long list of foods that reduce inflammation and decide which foods might be easy for you to incorporate more of into your diet. If it is a fresh fruit or vegetable, it is most likely anti-inflammatory.

- ☐ Focus on reducing the inflammation in your body through the foods that you are eating. Keep handy anti-inflammatory foods around your house. Avocados are a food that I always keep stocked in our house. We put them in our smoothies, add them to our coconut wrap breakfast burritos and tacos, eat them plain, and we even use them to make chocolate pudding for the kids. They are convenient for so many dishes.

- [ ] Consider taking an omega-3 supplement to help balance your ratio of omega-6 and omega-3 fatty acids.

- [ ] Try an elimination diet to find food intolerances that may be causing local or systemic inflammation in your body.

MODEL IT.

- [ ] Choose your foods wisely and with intention and your children will learn to do the same. When you start feeling more energetic and healthy, you are sure to demonstrate the powerful impact of quality food to your family.

TEACH IT.

- [ ] Teach your kids about inflammation and its negative effects on the body. We use language that our kids can understand, like how our bellies or muscles feel swollen and tired inside from certain foods. When we eat anti-inflammatory foods, we talk to the kids about our bellies and muscles feeling energetic and strong and that these foods protect us from getting sick.

- [ ] Educate your kids on pro-inflammatory and anti-inflammatory foods. Encourage them to notice inflammatory symptoms in their bodies when they eat pro-inflammatory foods.

- [ ] Teach your family about the optimal omega-6 and omega-3 fatty acid ratio of 2:1, and inform them about the benefits of omega-3 supplementation and limiting foods that contain high levels of omega-6 fatty acids.

16

Organic, Grass-Fed, and Other Food Labels

There are enough health claims and health labels on foods these days to make our heads spin. At the very least, we're sure to be confused and uncertain about what is truly healthy and what is simply a marketing gimmick. How do we know what sources of information or what health claims to trust? If we are not clear about what labels mean we can easily be misled into buying foods that may, in fact, be unhealthy options. (It says "gluten-free," so it must be okay!) Alternately, we may unknowingly miss the opportunity to buy foods that are healthier for our bodies. Each of us values different qualities and characteristics in the foods that we buy, including the effect of the item's production on the environment and the treatment of animals. Therefore, we all will make our own priorities regarding which labels are most meaningful and helpful in identifying products we want to consume. But regardless of our different values, improving our understanding of what the labels actually mean, or don't mean, is an important step in order to align our values with our purchases. The following information is intended to inform you about the differences between labels and health claims so you can balance your values, your health, and even your bank account.

Organic

Organic this! Organic that! It is more expensive, but is it really better? Certainly a product that is labeled organic does not mean that it is a healthy option, but generally speaking organic foods do seem to offer a variety of advantages over their equivalent conventional alternatives. Many of us are deterred from organic foods due to their cost, but there are reasons why organic food is more expensive. For one, organic farming can be more labor intensive. Second, maintaining organic certification can be expensive. Third, organic feed for animals can cost twice as much as conventional feed. Fourth, organic farms are often smaller than conventional farms, which means fixed costs and overhead must be distributed across smaller product volumes. And finally, most organic farms are too small to receive government subsidies. As a general rule, smaller operations and higher quality products cost more. The inverse of this rule is exactly why the conventional, or non-organic, practices came into being. They presented efficiency and cost benefits. The good news is that trends are showing that as more people purchase organic products, operations are growing and spreading, and the prices are coming down.[1] In addition, as demands increase grocers start to offer a wider variety of organic products.

Who wants to spend more money if it's not well justified? Let's review what makes organic foods different than conventional products. First, organic crops must be grown in "safe soil." Farmers are not allowed to use synthetic pesticides, genetically modified organisms (GMOs), petroleum-based fertilizers, or sewage sludge-based fertilizers (solids left over at the end of the sewage treatment process)—these conventional practices have been criticized for causing inflammation, cancer, and disease in humans.[2] Animals raised organically (for meat, dairy, and eggs) must have access to the outdoors and be given organic, non-GMO feed, and are not allowed to be given antibiotics, growth hormones, animal by-products or medications in the absence of illness.[3]

The question still remains whether there is a significant nutritional difference between organic and conventional foods. Because of their strict standards, organic foods are said to provide a variety of subsequent health benefits. Some studies have shown that organic foods have a higher concentration of nutrients, including antioxidants, vitamins, and minerals than their conventionally grown counterparts. One study found that organic produce contained at least twice the nutritional mineral content found in conventionally raised supermarket produce. Other studies have shown that organic produce have higher amounts of antioxidants.[4] However, some studies have shown that there is no strong evidence that organic foods are significantly more nutritious than conventional produce. The verdict is still out, but my anecdotal experience makes me believe that the rich, dark colors that are a signature of organic produce contain more luscious micronutrients than their pale conventional competitors. Similarly, many organic products seem to have much more flavor than their conventional counterparts.

Beyond the potential nutritional benefits of organic foods there are many other reasons why organic options may be preferable to their conventional counterparts, whether for our food, our body, or our world. The following are some of those benefits:[5]

Organic food is often fresher: Fresh food tastes better because it is harvested closer to its natural ripening date. Organic food is usually fresher because it doesn't contain added preservatives that make it last longer. You might notice that your organic produce doesn't last as long as conventional produce. Despite the inconvenience of shorter shelf life, the fact that organic foods degrade within a normal period of time is a good sign that the food is less altered (whether preserved, genetically modified, or harvested too early) and probably better for us.

Organic produce contains fewer pesticides, herbicides, and fungicides. In organic farming, only restricted uses of pesticides are permitted; crops are grown with natural fertilizers (manure and compost), weeds are controlled naturally (crop rotation, hand-weeding, mulching, and tilling), and insects are controlled using natural methods (birds, good insects, traps).[6] Synthetic chemicals are widely used in conventional agriculture and residues remain on the food we eat, and pollutants spread in the air and soil. Many synthetic pesticide ingredients have been found to cause cancer, inflammation, chronic illness, brain and nervous system toxicity, blood disorders, and hormonal dysregulation. Whether natural pesticides used in organic farming are harmful to our health is currently a debated topic. The National Academy of Sciences states, "By the time the average child is a year old, she will have received the acceptable lifetime doses of eight pesticides from twenty commonly eaten foods." Just to be clear, organic does not equal "pesticide free." Their use is restricted or limited to an allowed list. Regardless, a study from Stanford University found that just 7 percent of organic foods were found to have traces of pesticides, compared to 38 percent of conventionally-farmed produce. Therefore, regardless of the practices used, it appears that reduced amounts of pesticides are passed on to us when we eat organic produce. Of note, farmers working with conventionally grown produce are themselves exposed to heavy amounts of these chemicals and pesticides and are being diagnosed with cancer at staggering rates.[7]

Other studies show that organic produce has far lower levels of dangerous heavy-metal residues such as aluminum, lead, and mercury.[8] It intuitively makes sense that the more natural soil that they are grown in would more likely provide rich nutrients to these foods. Conversely, it makes sense that artificial fertilizers, hormones, and other synthetic chemicals used in conventional food production might interfere (in known and unknown ways) with natural growing conditions.

Organically raised animals are NOT given antibiotics, growth hormones, or fed animal by-products. The use of antibiotics in conventional meat production creates antibiotic-resistant strains of bacteria. This means that when someone gets sick from these strains they will be less responsive to antibiotic treatment. In addition, organically raised animals are given more space to move around and access the outdoors, both of which help to keep the animals healthy. Growth hormones, given to increase production and profit, are routinely administered to conventionally raised animals and have been shown to cause early puberty and increased risk of cancer in the people who are exposed to these hormones in their diet. Growth hormones are not allowed in organic production. Lastly, conventionally raised animals are commonly fed dead (often sick) animals as a part of their diet. Organic takes a stance against this practice.

Organic food is GMO-free. Genetically Modified Organisms (GMOs) or genetically engineered (GE) foods are plants or animals whose DNA has been altered in ways that cannot occur in nature or in traditional crossbreeding. As mentioned in Chapter 8, these genetic modifications are often designed to make the plant resistant to pesticides or insecticides or to enhance a particular characteristic of the plant. It is a concern to many that our bodies have a difficult time processing and digesting GMOs because our digestive system may not recognize the substances as food. The body may in fact react to these foods as if they were foreign substances. The body's immune system then attacks these substances, resulting in chronic inflammation and eventually illness.[9] Not to mention, when the plant is bred to be resistant to pesticides and herbicides, it allows the farmer to use much higher doses of these chemicals than would be normally tolerated by the plant, increasing the overall pesticide and herbicide use in this and other countries.[10]

Organic farming is better for the environment. Studies have shown that organic farms have a lower environmental impact than conventional farms.[11] One of the main goals of organically grown and produced foods are to encourage environmentally friendly farming practices, cycling of natural resources, and growing foods without synthetic pesticides or chemical fertilizers. Organic farming practices aim to reduce pollution (air, water, soil), conserve water, reduce soil erosion, increase soil fertility, and use less energy when compared to conventional farming. Farming without synthetic

> pesticides is also better for nearby birds, insects, and small animals as well as people who live close to or work on the farms.[12] Interestingly, Nicaragua is leading the way in trying to make all of their produce organic, in large part due to this critical point that organic foods are better for the environment (and farm workers).[13] Go Nicaragua!

The use of the U.S.D.A. Organic label is voluntary, so even if a food producer follows organic practices he may not want to go through the rigorous process of becoming U.S.D.A. certified. This is especially true for smaller farming operations. Many farmers follow organic or better practices without obtaining the official certification. These farmers typically take pride in the quality of their products and will usually share their practices with the public. I encourage you to investigate the practices of local, small farms before assuming that a local product is not organic simply because it does not have the official organic certification. For instance, we used to purchase milk products from a small dairy farm called "Spokane Family Farm." I was intrigued with their milk (non-homogenized, low-vat pasteurized, and grass-fed) but noticed that it wasn't organic. I contacted the farm owner—incredibly easily, I must say—and she was delighted to talk about their practices and philosophies as well as the reasons that their product is not certified organic. She was obviously proud of the farm's unique and mindful approach to dairy quality. In the end, I learned that this product was not organic because of the value these farmers had in keeping their cows for a very long time (into old age, even past milk production years). At times they have to use antibiotics to treat an infected cow. Even though they wouldn't sell that treated cow's milk, U.S.D.A. Certified Organic requires that there are no antibiotics on the farm property. They weren't willing to practice under these regulations and allow one of their cows to suffer or die prematurely from an infection. That explanation worked for me, so we happily bought the milk for as long as it was available to us.

It is helpful to know which conventionally grown crops are likely to carry the highest levels of pesticide residues to help us decide which products are most important to buy organic. According to the Environmental Working Group, a nonprofit organization that analyzes the results of government pesticide testing in the U.S., the conventionally grown fruits and vegetables in the left column of the chart below were found to have the highest pesticide levels. In the right column, you will find fruits and vegetables that were found to have the lowest levels of pesticides. Many of these foods have thicker skin, which naturally protects them from pests, resulting in the need for less pesticides. If you are on a budget, you can comfortably buy these fruits and vegetables conventionally grown. You can get annual updates of this list from the Environmental Working Group.[14]

2015 Dirty Dozen™ Produce with the *most* pesticides (in order from most contaminated)		2015 Clean 15™ Produce with the *least* pesticides (in order from least contaminated)	
1.	Apples	1.	Avocados
2.	Peaches	2.	Sweet corn
3.	Nectarines	3.	Pineapples
4.	Strawberries	4.	Cabbage
5.	Grapes	5.	Sweet peas (frozen)
6.	Celery	6.	Onions
7.	Spinach	7.	Asparagus
8.	Sweet bell peppers	8.	Mangos
9.	Cucumber	9.	Papaya
10.	Cherry tomatoes	10.	Kiwi
11.	Snap peas	11.	Eggplant
12.	Potatoes	12.	Grapefruit
And…	Kale & Collard greens	13.	Cantaloupe
		14.	Cauliflower
		15.	Sweet potatoes

Rinsing fruits and vegetables with water reduces but does not eliminate pesticides. Peeling sometimes helps, but valuable nutrients often go into the compost pile with the skin. The best approach to dealing with pesticides is to wash and scrub *all* produce—including organic—thoroughly (I was taught to wash with a 10 percent acid solution like lemon or vinegar—10:1, water to acid ratio) and buy organic when possible.

Regulations governing meat and dairy farming vary from country to country. It is helpful to understand the U.S. regulations for organic meat and dairy in order to make the best decisions for your family. The following table was extracted from *helpguide.com,* a nonprofit organization that partners with Harvard Health Publications to make quality public health education more accessible.[15] In the U.S., the major differences in organic and conventional meat and dairy include:

Conventionally Raised Meat & Dairy	Organic Meat & Dairy
Typically are given antibiotics, hormones, and GMO feed that is grown with pesticides.	No antibiotics, hormones, or GMO feeds are given to animals.
Livestock are given growth hormones for faster growth.	Livestock are given all organic feed.
Antibiotics and medications are used to prevent livestock disease.	Disease is prevented with natural methods such as clean housing, rotational grazing, and a healthy diet.
Livestock may or may not have access to the outdoors.	Livestock and milk cows must graze on pasture for at least four months per year, while chickens must have freedom of movement, fresh air, direct sunlight, and access to the outdoors.

Also extracted from *helpguide.org,* the United States Department of Agriculture permits the following to be fed to conventionally produced animals:

Animal	Conventional Feed
Dairy Cows	Antibiotics, pig and chicken by-products, growth hormones, pesticides, and sewage sludge.
Beef Cows	Antibiotics, pig and chicken by-products, steroids, growth hormones, pesticides, and sewage sludge.
Pigs	Antibiotics, animal by-products, pesticides, sewage sludge, and arsenic-based drugs (growth hormones are prohibited).
Broiler Chickens	Antibiotics, animal by-products, pesticides, sewage sludge, and arsenic-based drugs (growth hormones are prohibited).
Egg-Laying Hens	Antibiotics, animal by-products, pesticides, sewage sludge, and arsenic-based drugs.

Yes, organic food is often more expensive than conventionally grown food. But if you set some priorities, it may be possible to purchase organic food when it counts and still stay within your food budget. Purchase the organic versions of the foods you eat the most and those that have the highest pesticide levels or other disadvantages when conventionally grown. We can also save a bit of money if we buy in season. Fruits and vegetables are cheapest and freshest in season.

Remember that organic doesn't always equal healthy. Junk food can just as easily be made using organic ingredients. Making junk food sound healthy is a common marketing ploy in the food industry, but organic baked goods, desserts, and snacks are usually still very high in sugar, salt, unhealthy fat, or nutrient-deficient calories. So, don't be fooled—it pays to read food labels carefully.

Health Food Labels

The "U.S.D.A. Certified Organic" label is the most regulated certification for meat products, but we often see other certification labels on these food products. In order to make informed choices, it is helpful to understand what some of these terms mean. The top three labels listed are the most regulated.

U.S.D.A. Certified Organic

Foods are regulated by federal guidelines addressing soil quality, husbandry practices, pest and weed control, and use of additives. For produce, farmers use natural substances and physical, mechanical, or biological-based practices. Farmers are not allowed to use genetically modified crops. For meat, regulations require that animals are raised in living conditions accommodating their natural behaviors, fed 100 percent organic feed and forage, and not administered antibiotics or hormones. For multi-ingredient foods, regulations prohibit artificial preservatives, colors, or flavors and require that the ingredients be organic. There are three levels of organic claims on food labels:

1. *100% Organic Certified:* Products that are completely organic or made of only organic ingredients qualify for this claim and a U.S.D.A. Organic seal.
2. *Organic:* Products in which at least 95 percent of the ingredients are organic qualify for this claim and a U.S.D.A. Organic seal.
3. *Made with Organic Ingredients:* These are food products in which at least 70 percent of ingredients are certified organic and none of the ingredients are genetically modified. The U.S.D.A. Organic seal cannot be used, but "made with organic ingredients" may appear on its packaging.[16]

Grass-Fed

This term describes animals that are fed grass or hay and have continuous access to the outdoors. Cattle naturally eat grass, so cows tend to be healthier and leaner when fed this way. In addition, grass-fed beef has been shown to have more of the healthy omega-3 fatty acids than conventionally raised beef. However, if meat is labeled as grass-fed but not certified organic, the animal may have been raised on pasture that was exposed to or treated with synthetic pesticides or fertilizers. These animals may have been sent to a feed lot and fed grains (even if organic) before being butchered. Meat that is certified organic does not necessarily mean it is the healthiest option, as it could have been fed or finished with grain which has been shown to reduce the nutritional value of the meat. Only meat that is "grass finished" guarantees that the cattle consumed grass throughout its life. Some argue that grass-finished is more important than organic when it comes to beef. See the "Grass-Fed vs. Grain-Fed Animal Products" section below for more detailed information on grass-fed livestock.

Certified Humane, Animal Welfare Approved, and American Humane Certified (Poultry)

These are three different third-party certifiers for poultry. Certification is voluntary (companies choose whether or not to apply for certification) and ensures animals have ample space, shelter, gentle handling to limit stress, ample fresh water, and a diet without added antibiotics or hormones. Animals must be able to roam around without being confined to cages, crates, or tie stalls. Each certifier has various levels of certification and regulatory requirements.[17]

No Hormones Added or Hormone-Free

This term claims that animals are raised without the use of any added growth hormones. For beef and dairy products, this label can be indicative of healthier products, but by U.S. law poultry, veal calves, and pigs cannot be given hormones, so there is no need to pay extra for these products marketed with this label.[18]

Natural or All Natural

This label generally means "minimally processed" and that the product contains no artificial colors, artificial flavors, preservatives, or any other artificial ingredients in it. Animals can still be given antibiotics or growth enhancers and meat can be injected with salt, water, and other ingredients. For example, this term can be applied to all raw cuts of beef since they aren't processed. The natural label does not reflect how the animal was raised or fed which makes it fairly meaningless. There is no formal definition of the term "natural" from the F.D.A. or U.S.D.A., so be careful in interpreting this claim. The label must further explain the use of the term. Look for this additional labeling to better understand how that product defines "natural."[19]

Naturally Raised

This claim should be followed by a specific statement, such as "naturally raised without antibiotics or growth hormones" in order to obtain U.S.D.A. approval. Read different labels carefully to understand what naturally raised really means for the animal product you're buying.[20]

Free-Range or Free-Roaming (Poultry)

Broadly, this term means that the animals weren't confined to a cage and had access to the outdoors. There are no government-regulated standards for this claim, so it is difficult to know feeding and sheltering practices. Unfortunately, there are no requirements for the amount of time the animals spend outdoors or for the size of the outdoor space available. In addition the animals may or may not use the space provided, so the term may not necessarily represent any significant difference in the product. Beak cutting and forced molting through starvation are permitted. While it's difficult to tell exactly what free-range means on meat packaging, you can contact the producer directly for clarification.[21]

Cage-Free (Poultry)

The term means that egg-laying hens are not raised in cages. However, it does not necessarily mean they have access to the outdoors. Beak cutting and forced molting through starvation are permitted.[22]

Pasture-Raised (Poultry)

This label claims that the animals were not raised in confinement. Typically, pasture-raised hens are kept outdoors most of the year on a spacious pasture covered with living plants and kept indoors at night for protection. Again, there are no government-regulated standards for exactly how much time the animals spend outside or the size of the outdoor space available, so it can be misleading. Beak cutting and forced molting through starvation are permitted.[23]

Grass-Fed vs. Grain-Fed Animal Products

It makes sense that the quality of the food we eat is largely influenced by the quality of the food our food eats. Shedding light on the poor living conditions and feeding practices of the animals that we consume brings dire news to those who eat meat. The majority of the beef found in grocery stores comes from cattle that are fattened in large grain-feeding operations commonly referred to as feedlots. Although the cattle may spend the majority of their life on a pasture, they will spend their last months of life being "finished" in a feedlot. A cattle feedlot is populated by as many as one hundred thousand animals sharing the same space while they are fed grains that increase weight at a rate much faster than what can be obtained on pasture. Feedlots are crowded, filthy, and foul-smelling (to put it mildly). I can't help but imagine a human equivalent; being kept in a crowded room, walking around in excrement, and being fed nothing but cake and candy as I pack on the pounds. What type of physique and health do you think I'd have? Now picture what that same approach does to the body composition and health of your typical "corn finished" cow. The purpose of the feedlot is to quickly and efficiently increase weight (more weight equals more meat and more profit) and marbling—for flavor. But this extra weight and fat (marbling) come at the expense of the cow's health and well-being, which I, and many others, believe is transferred to us as we eat the meat.

It wasn't long ago that the beef industry began branding "corn-fed" beef as superior to all other forms of beef due to its tenderness and flavor. Cows fed corn develop well-marbled flesh which tastes great and was supposedly superior to more lean meats. The quick weight gain results and the economics of corn supply easily explain why this strategy made sense for the beef industry. Corn is likely the cheapest and most convenient food source. U.S. government corn subsidies can actually enable farmers to sell corn for less than what it costs to grow. And when it comes to industrial farming, cost and efficiency are king. Feedlots are able to cram thousands of cows together in feedlots where they are fattened up quickly on a mixture of corn and a slurry of other ingredients including liquefied fat, animal protein, synthetic estrogen, and antibiotics.[24] Although these methods maximize meat production, they also alter the nature of the meat. Corn-finished meat contains higher amounts of omega-6 fatty acids and less omega-3 fatty acids (often a ratio of 10-20:1), which throws off the balance of these two essential nutrients. Grass-finished beef, on the other hand, is leaner and contains a more balanced ratio of fatty acids. The ratio of omega-6 to omega-3 fatty acids for 100 percent grass fed (and finished) beef is 2-3:1, a perfect ratio for optimal health.[25]

Amazingly, corn is the cornerstone of the modern day feedlot strategy, despite the fact that a cow's digestive system has not evolved to digest it. Consequently, cows experience massive health problems due to all of the corn they are fed. To counteract the illnesses resulting from corn consumption, antibiotics are routinely required in order to keep the cattle healthy enough to survive. Recall that approximately 80 percent of the antibiotics sold in America are given to animals. To me the most disconcerting part of this series of events is the fact that most cattle are ill when they are butchered for our consumption. Another widely acknowledged side effect is that this practice greatly contributes to the evolution of new antibiotic-resistant "superbugs."

In addition to the corn-based diet and the use of antibiotics, the animals are also frequently injected with synthetic growth hormones such as estrogen which adds about forty to fifty pounds to the slaughter weight. These long-lasting chemicals end up in the meat we consume and also make their way into our waterways through the massive amounts of feedlot waste that escapes into the environment. These unhealthy and potentially inhumane farming operations create unhealthy animals that pass on health consequences to those of us who eat them.

On the flipside, is traditional pasture farming, wherein cows are raised on their natural diet of grasses in a low-stress environment. Feedlots manage thousands of head per day on a limited number of acres. Most ranchers run one cow per five to forty acres to ensure that one animal has adequate grass to graze. The results are healthy cows with no need for antibiotics or hormone supplements. In turn, their meat is healthier for us. Pasture-raised and finished grass-fed beef is leaner than grain-fed beef and higher in healthy omega- 3 fatty acids, CLAs, Vitamin E, and Beta Carotene.[26]

So, just because a piece of beef is certified organic does not mean it is healthier. Chances are that the cow was finished with corn, meaning it still has an unhealthy fat balance. Certified organic beef simply means the meat comes from animals that have not been treated with antibiotics or hormones and have been fed certified organic feed. There is nothing prohibiting the feeding of grain or corn to certified organic beef, unless the beef is labeled "Certified Organic Grass-Fed Beef."

Know Where Your Food Comes From

In this chapter, we have reviewed the criteria for organic, grass-fed, and other health labels as a step towards making better decisions about food quality. We can't have black and white thinking when assessing our food based on these labels—not all organic products are healthy, and being grass-fed does not mean you should eat excessive amounts of beef. There are certainly flaws and downsides to label-based production standards—they aren't perfect. Ideally, we would get to know the farmers and ranchers that supply our food and understand their food production practices. Unfortunately, this is not realistic for most of us. Therefore, a realistic goal is to move one step closer to being better informed and making better decisions. The more we learn about these topics the more ammo we have to make healthy decisions for our family.

☑ LIVE IT. MODEL IT. TEACH IT.

LIVE IT.

- [ ] Take time to clearly define your food values. Is organic important to you? What about cage-free eggs, or grass-fed meat? Only you can know what types of foods are important for you.

- [ ] Examine the value you put on quality of food versus price of food. Find the balance between cost and quality that works best for you and your financial situation and confidently make shopping decisions accordingly.

- [ ] Consider growing some of your own vegetables as a source of healthy food as well as to build the connection you and your family have to food. And get your hands into that microbe rich soil.

- [ ] Learn more about the production practices of the animal products that you consume. Make conscious decisions about what you value in quality, environmental impact, and animal welfare when choosing animal products and find products that adequately meet your values.

- [ ] Purchase produce locally when you are able and get to know the practices of your local farmers.

MODEL IT.

- [ ] You are teaching your children what to value and how to shop by what you pay attention to in the grocery store and what labels and foods they see in your house. They are learning a lifelong skill of how to make quality food decisions for themselves.

TEACH IT.

- ☐ Inform your children about the benefits and trade-offs of organic produce and meats.

- ☐ Help your family develop the ability to make balanced decisions regarding food purchases. For example, we went through a period of time when money was tight. I was grocery shopping with the boys and they wanted me to buy some bean chips. I told them that we weren't able to buy the bean chips because we had to be careful how we spent our money. "If we buy the chips we won't have the money to buy the kale we need for our ninja juice."

- ☐ Talk about conventionally raised animal products and how they impact our environment and our health.

- ☐ Teach your family about grass-fed beef and how important it is for livestock (just like us) to get chlorophyll and important omega-3 fats for them to be healthy and pass that health onto your family.

- ☐ Teach your kids that how we spend our money is equivalent to our voice in this world. If we want a healthy world for our children and grandchildren we confirm this by spending our money on products that promote that type of future.

17

Milk, Does it Do a Body Good?

My husband had what he describes as a mind-blowing awakening to milk while living in a small rural village in West Africa. Milk was a luxury food item for the Mandinka tribe that he lived with, as they were farmers not herders. But neighboring Fula tribes were herders and had access to daily milk. The first time he obtained some fresh milk he foolishly drank it immediately, assuming that it would quickly spoil in the hot African temperatures. He soon learned that whenever someone would get their hands on some milk, they would leave it in a covered bowl for a day or two, and then eat it sour. At first sight it looked repulsive. Thoughts of milk gone bad at home prevented him from trying the sour milk for months. But after repeatedly witnessing the enthusiasm saved for this treat, he eventually had to try this chunky, gooey slop. It was amazing. He claims that in the refrigerator-less bush, it was like getting ice cream. What he didn't realize until much later was that the reason our milk goes bad when it gets sour is due to the processing and pasteurization it goes through. Pure, raw milk right from the cow doesn't get rancid like our pasteurized milk. It gets sour (rich in probiotics) and is at its best flavor in this state. It turns out that the milk he was getting was extremely healthy compared to our processed milk. Raw, untreated milk from exclusively open range, grass-fed cattle with no exposure to pesticides, hormones, antibiotics, and genetically modified feed is not even a close relative to any of the milk you will find in the grocery store in the United States. This insight begs the question: What are the health implications of what we do to our milk after it leaves the cow?

The debate of whether or not cow's milk is a health food is a complicated and sometimes touchy subject. There is conflicting research and literature to prove and disprove its necessity in our diet. That makes the milk conversation confusing. I try not to subscribe fully one way or the other with dairy, as I think it is a choice that every family needs to make for themselves. That said, I have found that as I better understand milk and the dairy industry, I have been able to make decisions that I am comfortable with for my family. The American Dairy Board has done an effective job marketing dairy products and educating us about the benefits of cow's milk. I will not rehash the benefits of milk that most of us have subscribed to for most of our lives. Instead, I will outline some of the concerns about modern pasteurized milk, some of the threats that dairy products may pose to our health, and some of the potential benefits of raw milk. This information has ultimately led to my family limiting dairy intake, but you may find different solutions for your family as you explore this process.

To begin, of interest is the estimated 60 percent of the world's population that is unable to digest pasteurized milk well.[1] In fact, some researchers believe that being able to digest milk beyond infancy is actually abnormal. Milk is a common allergen (the most common in the U.S., in fact) and often triggers an inflammatory response in many individuals, causing stomach distress, allergies, asthma, eczema, ear infections, constipation, diarrhea, gas, skin rashes, and acne—yes, acne! I have known many people who have successfully eliminated dairy to control their acne or other types of inflammatory symptoms, including our second son (in his case dairy was eliminated along with other foods). This evidence certainly brings to question the appropriateness of our consumption of milk. But let's look deeper at the various issues.

Is Cow Milk Just For Cows?

One argument that some make against consuming milk products is the fact that humans are consuming a product that, by nature's standards, evolved for a baby cow. Biologically speaking, the milk of different mammals varies considerably in its composition. For example, the milk of goats, elephants, humans, cows, camels, wolves, and walruses show marked differences in their content of fats, proteins, sugars, and minerals. Each evolved to provide the optimum nutrition to the specific young of each respective species. The fact that cow's milk did not evolve for human consumption may be why pasteurized cow milk is the number one allergic food in this country. In general, most animals are exclusively "breast-fed" until they have tripled their birth weight, which in human infants occurs around the age of one year. Except for the domestic cat, humans are the only mammalian species that consumes milk past the weaning period.[2] Whether consuming the milk of another species is healthy or not is up for debate. Some argue convincingly that raw and cultured dairy products from healthy grass-fed cows can be extremely healthy for humans. As we leave that question to future research, or Fula tribal insights, let's examine some of the factors about milk for which we do have more information.

Cattle Feeding Practices

There are concerns about modern feeding methods that directly impact the effect that milk has on our health. Cows evolved eating grass. But in recent times their diet has been altered significantly to include primarily high-protein, soy- and corn-based feeds, as well as hormones and vitamins, to boost milk production. This diet, along with confined living conditions, tends to make the cows ill. Consequently, these cows are given antibiotics. In addition, this unnatural diet changes the nutritional makeup of the milk. Similar to the difference between grain-fed and grass-fed beef, the conventional dairy products that we consume are nutritionally completely different than the unaltered Fula milk in Africa. When buying U.S.D.A. Certified Organic milk we know that the cows have not been given any antibiotics, and they are required to have some access to pasture, though this doesn't necessarily mean they have been raised on a grass-only diet. Therefore, if we are going to consume milk and milk products, a good starting point would be to look for organic and grass-only fed dairy.

The use of rBGH (Recombinant Bovine Growth Hormone) by dairy farmers to increase milk production is another concern with milk. rBGH is a genetically modified artificial hormone that causes an increase in an insulin-like growth factor (IGF-1) which is found in the milk of treated cows. IGF-1 survives milk pasteurization and human intestinal digestion. It can be directly absorbed into the human bloodstream, particularly in infants. IGF-1 has been shown to promote the transformation of human breast cells into cancerous forms. IGF-1 also supports growth of already cancerous breast and colon cancer cells, advancing their progression and invasiveness. We absorb the rBGH directly from the milk which can actually cause further IGF-1 production by our own cells. rBGH also results in increased mastitis (breast infections) in cows, for which they must receive additional antibiotics. When purchasing milk, ensure that the milk is free from rBGH. Certified Organic dairy is required to be free from rBGH.[3]

Pasteurization and Processing

Modern milk sold in the grocery store undergoes significant processing from the time it is milked from the cow to the time it lands on the shelf at the store. Milk is usually "ultra-pasteurized." This means that the milk is heated to high temperatures in order to kill harmful bacteria. Unfortunately this process also ends up destroying the essential enzymes needed for us to absorb the available nutrients in milk. Our pancreas often cannot produce the enzymes needed to digest the milk, resulting in over-stressing of the pancreas. Similarly pasteurization kills much of the healthy bacteria that aids in digestion of milk and nurtures our intestinal microbiome. Pasteurization is the reason that our milk gets rancid instead of simply turning sour like the Fulas' milk. The bacteria that are killed in the pasteurization process are needed to ferment the milk (just like with yogurt) and make it sour and full of beneficial probiotics.

Another stage of typical milk processing is homogenization. The butterfat in milk naturally separates to the top. In the homogenization process the fat globules are shaken up into such small shards that they are distributed evenly throughout the milk, providing a smooth and consistent texture. It has been suspected that homogenized milk boosts the absorbability of an enzyme in milk called xanthine oxidase, which increases disease-promoting inflammatory processes associated with heart disease, diabetes, allergies, and other chronic disorders. There is no clear evidence that homogenization is good or bad; however, it is worth noting simply because the process does change the original form of the food. History shows us that nature does a much better job at designing foods than we do.

Even more concerning is the process of removing butterfat to make skim milk or low-fat milk. It may come as a surprise based on what we've been told for years, but skim milk (including 1 percent and 2 percent) is not a healthier choice than whole milk. Skim milk is what remains after the cream has been removed in a separator. Unfortunately, the cream is where we find the healthy enzymes and fat-soluble vitamins. Because the vitamins are removed with the cream, the milk is often fortified with synthetic vitamins (such as synthetic Vitamin D, which has raised concerns about toxicity to the liver) in an attempt to add back what has been lost. Removing the fat in milk brings about other complications as well. Processors must go to great lengths to replace the body or creamy texture of milk by working in various food additives. In the case of low-fat or skim milk, that usually means adding powdered milk. Powdered milk contains oxidized cholesterol, the harmful form of cholesterol. To overcome this problem, companies sometimes compensate by adding antioxidants. You can see the problematic chain effect that results from the desire to make milk "fat-free." Have you ever looked at the ingredient labels of some individual milk cartons (like those served with school lunches, for example)? You may be amazed to notice the amount of sugar that can be added to milk. It's a shame what we do to a product that was originally a simple whole food. If you are going to drink milk, it is best to consume the real thing and avoid processed forms, including skim and low-fat.[4]

Raw Milk

Raw milk is neither pasteurized nor homogenized, instead coming straight from the cow without modification or processing. This is the milk my husband fell in love with in Africa. Raw milk has been found to provide many health benefits, including being tolerated by most people who are otherwise (in the case of pasteurized milk) dairy intolerant. It has been shown to provide a boost in healthy bacteria to the GI tract, be a source of conjugated linoleic acid (a cancer fighter), and have a healthy omega-3 and omega-6 balance. Despite this evidence, the fear over bacterial infection has caused widespread concern by public health agencies. Public health officials and the National Dairy Council have worked together in the United States to make it very difficult to obtain fresh, raw dairy products. Nevertheless, raw milk can be found with a little effort. In some states, you can buy raw milk directly from farmers. In other states you can purchase a "share" of a cow, essentially allowing you to "own" your own cow—and therefore its milk. There are also companies that pasteurize their milk at low temperatures, in order to preserve much of the bacteria that enhance our bodies' ability to digest it. We have purchased Spokane Family Farm milk in the past and have loved it. Other options seem to eliminate some of the problems while retaining others. For example, whole, non-homogenized milk from organic or grass-fed cows, but still pasteurized, is available in many gourmet shops and health food stores. There may not be an absolute wrong or right answer in selecting dairy products, but understanding the differences moves us one step in the direction of making clear choices for our situations and families.

Milk, Calcium, and Bones

Because the U.S.D.A. has promoted milk as the primary source of calcium for bone health, you might be wondering what will happen to your bones and teeth if you stop consuming dairy. Calcium is currently at the center of one of nutrition's most contentious debates. Proponents of milk praise it as a primary source of calcium and a means to protect our bones from fractures. Critics say that there is actually little evidence that high intake of calcium has more than a marginal effect on bone density and fracture prevention and that paying more attention to exercise and vitamin D may be more advantageous to the health of our bones.[5]

Many recent studies debate milk's ability to strengthen bones. Ironically, osteoporosis (thinning of the bones) is highest in those countries that consume the highest amount of calcium from animal-based sources—milk.[6] The Twelve-Year Nurse Study at Harvard University followed seventy-eight thousand nurses over twelve years and found that those who drank two or more glasses of milk per day had twice the risk of hip fractures than those who drank a glass or less a week. Other large-scale studies have validated that high calcium intake doubles the risk of hip fractures. How could this be? We have been taught for decades that consuming calcium (in the form of milk) strengthens our bones. One reason this theory may not be true is that cow's milk is rich in phosphorous which can combine with calcium and actually prevent us from absorbing most of the calcium. Another possibility could be that milk protein accelerates calcium excretion from the blood through the kidneys. One of the last theories, which gave me a big "ah-ha" moment, is related to our body's pH level. Our bodies have to maintain a consistent pH balance, and most foods either make our bodies more acidic or more alkaline. Milk is claimed to increase acidity in the body. One of the ways our body then rebalances our pH is by pulling alkaline minerals from our bones to balance the overly acidic state it finds itself in. Therefore, consuming milk, at least in the absence of significant amounts of alkaline-inducing foods (mainly vegetables), could actually reduce rather than increase the strength of our bones.[7]

These arguments and research studies certainly fuel the debate as to whether or not milk strengthens or weakens our bones. However, what we do know is that our bodies require many nutrients working together for good bone health, including magnesium, phosphorus, boron, copper, manganese, zinc, vitamins C, D, K, B6, and folic acid.[8] In addition, our bones need protein to build collagen and fats for the absorption of Vitamin D. And calcium can only be absorbed with adequate amounts of Vitamin D. Bone health is complicated and unlikely to be significantly altered by one lifestyle decision (drinking or not drinking milk). Therefore, I suggest another, better understood strategy to strengthen and manage bone health. Instead of focusing on milk as the primary source for optimal bone health, if we focus on eating real foods, especially a variety of fruits and vegetables, our bones will get the nutrients they need. Although calcium is clearly not the only factor relevant to bone health, it is one of the most abundant minerals in the human body. We associate it with bone and tooth health, but it is also important for muscle development, healthy blood pressure, and skin health. There are many foods that are just as high—if not higher—in calcium than dairy products. Including the following recommendations into our diet and lifestyle will help us reap the many benefits of calcium regardless of whether we consume dairy products. And by the way, the amount of vitamin D that is needed to absorb the calcium we need is obtained by simply getting ten to fifteen minutes of direct sunshine exposure (without sunscreen) per day.

- *Five to seven vegetables per day (especially leafy greens like kale, watercress, and collard greens. Second to leafy greens in high calcium content is broccoli.)*
- *Fish with bones (canned sardines or salmon)*
- *Soup stocks (preferably homemade with organic bones)*
- *Sunflower and pumpkin seeds*
- *Nuts (almonds have the highest amount of calcium per serving out of all tree nuts)*
- *Whole grains in modest amounts*
- *Beans (soaking beans overnight in water is important to decrease the phytic acid content which will allow for optimal absorption of minerals)*
- *Naturally raised animal protein (like grass-fed and -finished beef)*
- *Olive oil*
- *Flaxseed*
- *Regular exercise*
- *Avoiding or minimizing refined sugars, honey, and white flour (including pasta, bread, muffins, and most baked desserts) because these all can contribute to acidic pH levels that subsequently leach minerals from your bones*[9]

Because of the conflicting studies and advice, whether or not to consume dairy can be a confusing choice. Milk has been such a cornerstone of our food culture for so long. Experiment with dairy to see what works best for your family. Remember, roughly 60 percent of people around the world are unable to digest pasteurized milk well. Many of us may be drinking milk and not realizing that we would feel and function a lot better without it. Earlier we reviewed dairy's ability to cause many local and systemic reactions in the body like acne, eczema, irregular stools, irritability, even asthma. It can contribute to any of the symptoms of leaky gut and food sensitivities. Therefore, many of us would likely benefit from either eliminating or significantly reducing conventional milk consumption in our diets. If you are interested, start by decreasing or eliminating dairy for several weeks and reevaluate how you feel after that time. If you decide to eliminate all dairy, remember that skim milk and Lact-Aid milk, cheese, yogurt, and ice cream should also be eliminated. When you reintroduce milk back into your diet after two to three weeks you will likely notice uncomfortable symptoms more acutely at that time, which will be a key indicator of your level of tolerance for milk.

☑ LIVE IT. MODEL IT. TEACH IT.

LIVE IT.

- ☐ Decide for yourself if dairy is a good source of nutrition for your family, and if so, decide which forms align with your values and philosophy.

- ☐ Experiment with cutting milk out of your diet for a test period. Initially you may think that you can't live without dairy, but you may end up being surprised how easy it is with the many milk substitutes available. Take careful note of how you feel while consuming and while avoiding dairy. Our family now uses coconut milk and almond milk (which contains 50 percent more calcium than milk) and we don't even miss cow's milk anymore. Two years ago when we eliminated milk from our daily diet, I thought we wouldn't survive, and I would have no idea how to cook. Now, I barely think about it. Lifestyle changes can seem scary because of the unknown and the steep learning curve, but the effects on our health are often worth it.

MODEL IT.

- [ ] If you do have an undesirable reaction to dairy, see it as an opportunity to demonstrate to your children what it looks like to listen to your body and be open to lifestyle changes, especially changes that may seem initially intimidating. What a gift for your children to see that we don't have to blindly follow convention when our body tells us otherwise, but rather that we can listen to ourselves and make decisions based on what is best for us.

TEACH IT.

- [ ] Teach your children that there is debate and controversy regarding dairy. Challenge your family to do a dairy elimination trial and document how everyone responds.

- [ ] Help your children connect fatigue, acne, skin issues, constipation, and diarrhea with potential food allergies and sensitivities and empower them to evaluate their own needs and make lifestyle decisions based on how they feel and how their body reacts.

18

What's the Deal With Wheat?

As our family began to minimize the amount of processed sugars and grains in the early stages of our exploration with improving our diets, we naturally began to avoid most breads and other sources of wheat. But we still ate whole grain wheat or sprouted grain wheat bread, and didn't worry too much about periodic whole wheat sandwiches and other common wheat-based foods. During this time we continued to hear many personal stories from friends who had eliminated wheat, often motivated by a relative who may have had a serious sensitivity to wheat, even celiac disease. These friends seemed to consistently experience significant health improvements, many times in very unexpected ways. Their stories piqued our interest but still did not convince us to go cold turkey on the "golden waves of grain."

Our family's first introduction to wheat elimination came when a naturopath recommended that we eliminate wheat, dairy, and corn from our son's diet in order to heal his inflamed digestive system. We eliminated these foods from his diet and began to nurture his microbiome with probiotics. To our amazement and joy, he soon began to normalize with healthy bowel movements, and his behavioral challenges improved drastically. Certainly this was no double-blind scientific experiment, but after trying to resolve this problem for so long, we suspected even more strongly that eliminating wheat could be beneficial for his health.

Our second significant experience came from an experiment my husband conducted after being inspired by Dr. William Davis' book *Wheat Belly.* Just before Thanksgiving 2013, he decided to try eliminating wheat completely. He didn't have specific symptoms in mind that he wanted to address but was simply curious about the associations between wheat and other ailments. It seemed harmless, if not prudent, to at least give it a try. Thanksgiving Day provided the first piece of evidence—and test of will power—that this was a good move. My husband avoided all wheat products and refined sugars (which he already avoided as much as possible) during the entire holiday and found that not once did he have the accustomed bloated, uncomfortable, fall-down-on-the-couch and pass-out-during-football -games feeling. He ate amply, as he always does at Thanksgiving but to his delight felt fantastic the whole weekend. This experience gave him the motivation to keep going with the wheat prohibition. In time he noted other benefits. What had been regular bouts of constipation during an entire lifetime, simply went away. This wasn't even really something he had considered a problem, but rather just the way his body worked. He experienced less gas, less grogginess after meals, and best of all he stopped feeling bloated after meals. As our personal experiences continued to validate what we were learning about the suspected impacts of gluten, and wheat in particular, on our bodies' systems, we felt we had enough evidence to decide to take wheat out of our family diet. Despite the conflicting messages in the research, media, and government recommendations, we felt that it couldn't hurt.

Is Gluten-Free Just a Fad?

At the extreme end of the spectrum, some people can have severe responses to the gluten in wheat, leading to intestinal bleeding. This autoimmune response to gluten is what's referred to as celiac disease. Gluten is a protein found in wheat, barley, and rye (and sometimes in oats). When people with celiac disease eat foods containing gluten, their immune system responds by damaging a particular part of their small intestine that allows nutrients from food to be absorbed directly into the bloodstream. About one in 133 people in the United States have celiac disease, and it is estimated that 80 percent of people with celiac disease are undiagnosed.[1] Celiac disease is a very severe condition, and absolute avoidance of gluten is necessary. But why should the other 132 of us consider avoiding wheat? Neither my son nor my husband has celiac disease. It turns out that, like many health issues, reactions to gluten exist on a continuum. Celiac disease may be the extreme end of the spectrum, but many of us experience significant health problems resulting from the consumption of gluten. In fact, many health experts claim that most people have issues with gluten, stating that in many cases the symptoms are simply not recognized because they are not severe, there is no diagnosis of any ailment, or no common test that can prove a problem.

The Impact of Wheat in the Body

How can gluten sensitivity be explained? "Bread has been around for thousands of years! It doesn't make sense for so many people to claim to be gluten intolerant!" I hear versions of this statement regularly when I tell people that my family tries to avoid gluten. And it's truly a great question. In fact, the expansion of modern civilization has been linked to agricultural developments greatly based on wheat production. So, how could Jesus' bread be important enough to become a symbol of Jesus himself, while today many medical experts suggest that its consumption should be minimized or avoided? One of the explanations is the fact that Jesus' wheat is genetically about as different from our wheat as humans are to chimpanzees. Through the natural process of seed selection and hybridization, the actual wheat grain has been changed so dramatically, and more importantly, so quickly, that some believe our body does not even recognize it as a food. Wheat has changed dramatically during even the short lifetimes of most readers of this book. The modern wheat crop is not the same wheat that even our grandparents ate. Therefore, many argue, it is also not recognizable to our digestive system. If wheat is not recognized in our digestive tract it can more easily trigger an immune response. Recall that the immune system's job is to protect us from foreign or offending substances; this includes foods that it doesn't recognize. The end result is inflammation in many parts of the body. When consumed on a regular basis we experience chronic inflammation (see Chapter 3) as our body constantly tries to protect us from this foreign substance.[2] No one is at fault here. We have simply wanted to make a better quality, more useful grain, using less water, land, time, and fertilizer.

A second explanation, or potential contributing factor, to our ever growing sensitivity to wheat, has been explained by the dire state of the gut health of most Americans. As discussed in Chapter 11, more and more evidence is pointing to the importance of our microbiome to our health and our ability to break down and utilize foods. A healthy microbiome has the tools it needs to break down, absorb and utilize, or filter and eliminate, a wide variety of food and non-food substances. Because Americans tend to have a diminished gut microbiome due to the evolution of our largely unhealthy diets, we are unable to process the extremely difficult-to-digest gliadin protein in gluten.

Regardless of the explanations for widespread gluten sensitivity, many correlations between wheat/gluten and adverse health conditions have been observed. Dr. William Davis, in his book *Wheat Belly,* suggests that gluten sensitivity can be a factor in dozens of conditions ranging from Irritable Bowel Syndrome to Alzheimer's disease to skin disease and acne. In addition, the symptoms of gluten intolerance are not just physical. Davis explains how gliadin, a protein found within gluten, breaks down in the body into a substance called gluteomorphin, an opioid peptide that passes into the brain and disrupts brain function. There is evidence that the opioid receptors in the brain react to wheat as they would to heroin or other opioid drugs. Therefore, gluteomorphin may be the reason why wheat products have been shown to be addictive for many people.[3] Similarly, David Perlmutter's book *Grain Brain* highlights the significant effect that gluten has on brain function and neurological disorders, including being a significant contributing factor for dementia. Perlmutter cites seemingly miraculous neurological transformations experienced by severely debilitated patients when they simply eliminated gluten from their diets. Between the evidence presented by Davis and Perlmutter, it appears that if you happen to suffer from any sort of symptom, major or minor, whose cause has not been identified, it may be worth doing a "gluten free" experiment on yourself.[4]

If the evidence presented so far seems too far-fetched, simply looking at the glycemic index of wheat may be of interest. As a reminder, a food's glycemic index is the rate at which it is converted to sugar in the blood stream, as a comparison to pure glucose which has a glycemic index of one hundred. Foods with a high glycemic index or glycemic load have been shown to contribute to blood sugar and insulin spikes, which result in more calories being converted to fat in your body and an increase in cellular inflammation. Over time this can lead to type 2 diabetes and many other health conditions (see Chapter 9). The glycemic index of high-fructose corn syrup and sucrose (granulated table sugar) average about seventy-three and sixty-eight respectively. The glycemic index for wheat flour (white and whole wheat) averages between seventy-one and seventy-three. In regards to blood glucose levels, eating wheat bread is worse than eating straight table sugar.[5]

Pulverized Grains

Consuming "whole grain" wheat is frequently considered healthy and often promoted (even by the U.S. government). This claim may be misleading in the context of processed "whole grains," the form in which most of us encounter whole grains in the grocery store. Grains, including whole wheat, found in breads and pastries, as well as many supposed health foods and crackers, are pulverized grains. When grains are pulverized they are broken into fine pieces (flour) that become high on the glycemic index and have less nutritional value. The outer shell of the whole grain normally slows down sugar absorption from the grain as the digestive system has to work to penetrate and break it down. Once this shell is pulverized the resulting flour is now quickly absorbed by the body and turned into sugar. Pulverized grains are not optimal for our body; they wreak havoc on our blood sugar and insulin levels, waist line, and inflammatory markers.[6] You may or may not have felt suspicious the last time you read the claim for "Healthy Whole Grains" on the label of your favorite sugared cereal, but also beware of the same claim being made for breads, bagels, so-called "healthy" cereals, and other products.

Experimenting With Gluten-Free

Whether you are the type of person that responds to in-depth research data or the type that is inspired by the anecdotes of a dear friend, you should be able to find the inspiration to, at a minimum, think about wheat consumption in your family and perhaps try your own experiment. In the end all of our bodies are unique and respond differently to different foods and substances. Trusting your body and the experiments you subject it to will be the ultimate guide. Some of us will find that going completely gluten-free is the right answer, like my husband. Some, like me, will find that eliminating gluten the majority of the time is helpful but will allow themselves to indulge on certain occasions. For instance, most of the time I am gluten-free, but when it comes to the mouth-watering fresh bagel sandwich from our local bakery, I will occasionally indulge in a wheat-filled piece of heaven. Of course, many places, even bakeries, will accommodate gluten-free lifestyles by providing options that avoid wheat products—like the savory *Paleo Platter* at our local bakery that is void of baked goods altogether.

Now, if you are convinced in theory to even consider a new gluten-free lifestyle, you might be imagining what an impossible challenge it would be to eliminate wheat from your diet. Think of all our standard cultural landmarks: pizza, sandwiches, cereals, pasta, donuts, cakes, etc. But notice how most of those foods are made of refined carbohydrates and often full of sugar, foods whose negative health impacts have been highlighted throughout the book. Fortunately, as our view of what is health promoting has evolved, we have found that there are a vast amount of delicious foods to replace the standard wheat-based staples. It just takes a little creativity and thinking outside of the "box" until you get used to it. Be careful not to turn to easy and convenient "gluten-free" products in your attempts to avoid gluten. Many gluten-free products substitute gluten with similar starches like tapioca starch, rice flour, and potato starch which can be even higher on the glycemic index than wheat or sugar, causing high blood glucose levels and rapid insulin releases—of course contributing to cellular inflammation and weight gain. Not to mention many gluten-free products are highly processed and manufactured, full of ingredients and chemicals we don't need or want. In his book, Davis urges people to go *gluten free* without going "gluten-free." I agree. Fill your cart with vegetables and fruits and other foods that come from the earth, and limit your intake of foods in a package that claim to be healthy simply because they are "gluten-free." Remember "gluten-free" has become a money making industry (an over four billion dollar industry, in fact), and companies don't necessarily have our best interest at heart. I don't pay as much attention to our family being "gluten-free" as I do to our family eating real foods. They almost naturally go hand in hand.

I know many parents who have personally eliminated gluten from their diets yet struggle to get the rest of the family on board. I often hear about individuals who attempt this transition independently because their spouse and/or kids aren't interested in becoming gluten-free. I know some people who make multiple dishes to accommodate everyone's needs; for instance, preparing traditional spaghetti for the family and brown rice noodles for the gluten-free member(s). Or when converting to a gluten-free lifestyle it may be tempting to continue purchasing conventional cereal for the rest of the family while searching out gluten-free cereal for yourself. The potential problem with this perspective is that the "gluten-free" focus distracts us from the fact that both cereals are highly processed, manufactured, and full of sugar. Other family members may rightly perceive that there isn't a significant difference between the gluten-free option and what they eat. Why would they change? I think a paradigm shift with gluten-free eating is important when trying to get the whole family to eat the same foods. Instead of thinking about substituting gluten products with other refined grains simply to avoid the gluten, think about how you can replace these processed wheat foods with real (whole) foods. For example, we rarely use gluten-free noodles; we use spaghetti squash or shredded zucchini as noodles. We are not just *eliminating* gluten, we are *adding* a vegetable. We typically don't substitute gluten-free tortillas for wheat tortillas; we use either coconut wraps that are 100 percent coconut or Romaine lettuce for the wrap. Healthy gluten-free substitutes for breakfast cereal can include eggs and veggies, nut porridges, sautéed mushrooms, or green smoothies, for example. Notice how these alternatives are not just gluten-free but are real foods that are packed with vitamins, minerals, antioxidants, and phytonutrients. When we focus on real food substitutions the whole family benefits, even those that aren't interested in being "gluten-free."

Wheat Withdrawal

Some people experience withdrawal symptoms after eliminating wheat. Withdrawal symptoms can be uncomfortable, and some people think that their bodies must be telling them that they need wheat. The withdrawal symptoms are part of a transitional phase as your body tries to return to its normal state. Some people experience headaches, nausea, intense wheat cravings, bloating, constipation, fatigue, inability to exercise, or even feeling depressed. It is unfortunate that some individuals misinterpret these discomforts as their body's "need" for wheat, and they reintroduce wheat back into their diets. Be aware that these withdrawal symptoms generally resolve themselves within a week. Dr. Davis has many suggestions to support withdrawal symptoms from wheat on his blog *wheatbellyblog.com*. Try to hang in there through this potentially uncomfortable experience because it is your body healing from many years of wheat addiction and dependence.[7]

☑ LIVE IT. MODEL IT. TEACH IT.

LIVE IT.

- ☐ Whether you choose to reduce or eliminate wheat in your diet or not, keep in mind how processed and modified our modern wheat is.

- ☐ You may want to limit wheat or white flour as a first step. Maybe you feel like eating only sprouted wheat breads and tortillas (Ezekiel brand is in the freezer section of most modern grocery or health food stores) and cutting out highly refined crackers, cookies, pretzels, and other snack foods.

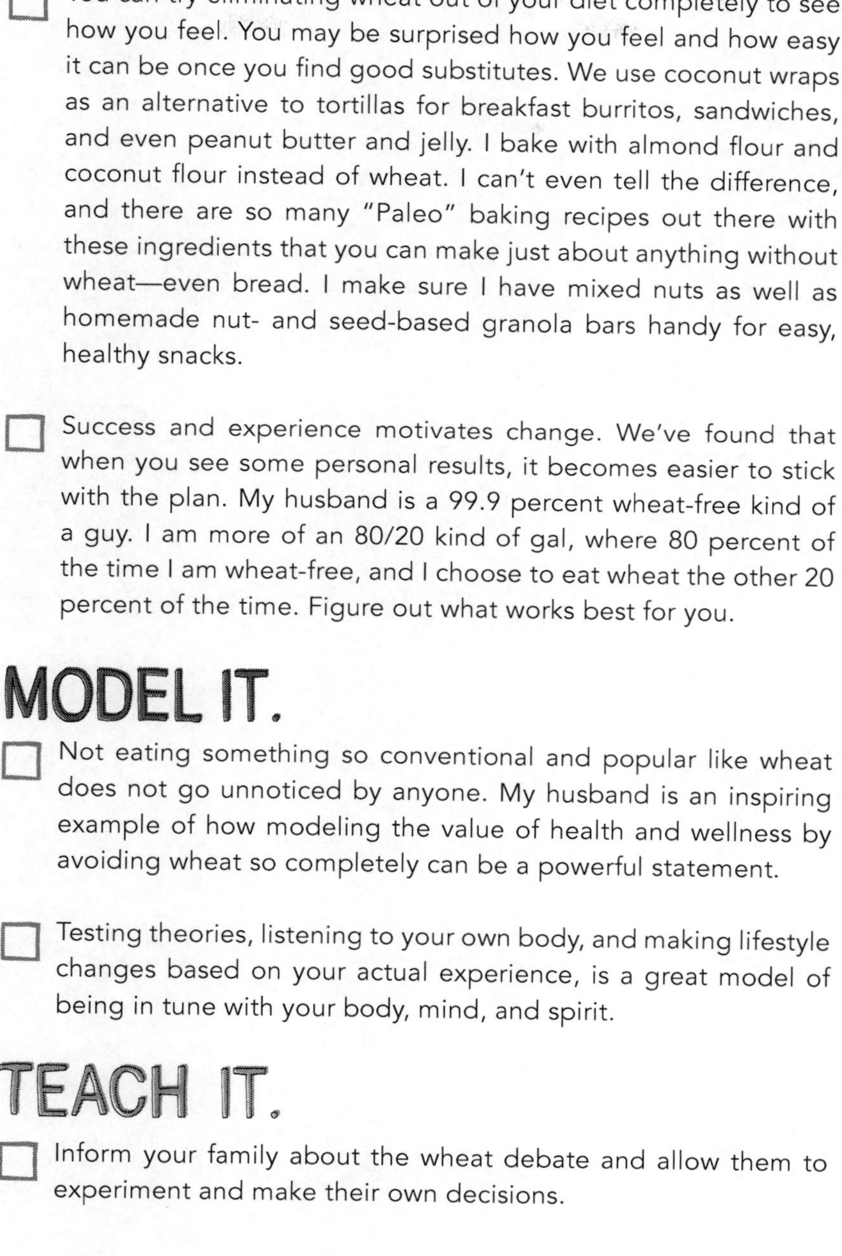

☐ You can try eliminating wheat out of your diet completely to see how you feel. You may be surprised how you feel and how easy it can be once you find good substitutes. We use coconut wraps as an alternative to tortillas for breakfast burritos, sandwiches, and even peanut butter and jelly. I bake with almond flour and coconut flour instead of wheat. I can't even tell the difference, and there are so many "Paleo" baking recipes out there with these ingredients that you can make just about anything without wheat—even bread. I make sure I have mixed nuts as well as homemade nut- and seed-based granola bars handy for easy, healthy snacks.

☐ Success and experience motivates change. We've found that when you see some personal results, it becomes easier to stick with the plan. My husband is a 99.9 percent wheat-free kind of a guy. I am more of an 80/20 kind of gal, where 80 percent of the time I am wheat-free, and I choose to eat wheat the other 20 percent of the time. Figure out what works best for you.

MODEL IT.

☐ Not eating something so conventional and popular like wheat does not go unnoticed by anyone. My husband is an inspiring example of how modeling the value of health and wellness by avoiding wheat so completely can be a powerful statement.

☐ Testing theories, listening to your own body, and making lifestyle changes based on your actual experience, is a great model of being in tune with your body, mind, and spirit.

TEACH IT.

☐ Inform your family about the wheat debate and allow them to experiment and make their own decisions.

- [ ] Ask your children how they feel after eating wheat products to teach them how to pay attention to their bodies' responses to foods.

- [ ] Show your family that wheat is an ingredient in a lot of food, and it is often highly processed and generally not a good choice for our bodies. Give them examples of packaging that claims to be "multi-grain" or "whole wheat" but whose ingredients reveal that the food is more refined and processed than the marketing claim lets on.

19

Super Health With Superfoods

"Superfood" seems like the new buzzword. I hear it everywhere. And, I must admit, I have begun to feel a little annoyed by the overuse of the term to refer to any and every healthy food. That said, there certainly are foods that provide an extraordinary amount of nutrients relative to the number of calories consumed. So while there is no generally accepted definition, superfoods are typically considered to be a class of the most potent, super-concentrated, and nutrient-rich foods on the planet. We've discussed the many benefits of green leafy vegetables in the context of the previous chapter themes, and they certainly should be the first superfood that we add to our diet. Collard, mustard, and turnip greens, kale, watercress, Swiss chard, and bok choy are some of the most nutrient dense greens available. The superfoods highlighted below are less common in most of our diets, but have a unique potential to accelerate health improvements. My goal is to treat green leafy vegetables as our family's staple for baseline health and the following foods as health boosters. Superfoods have the ability to tremendously increase the vital force and energy of our bodies and are a great way to optimize overall health by boosting the immune system, elevating serotonin production, enhancing sexuality, lowering inflammation, alkalizing the body, and many more potential benefits. Although including superfoods in our diet can super-size our health, we must remember that nothing is a quick fix. I have seen people become obsessed with superfoods thinking that they magically make us healthy. Superfoods are not magical in this way. Balance and variety are key elements to health, and we must always look at health in the whole picture context: considering both primary and secondary food elements.

Below are some of the more common superfoods. I recommend that you experiment with some or all of them to determine which are the best for your family—both in terms of needs and preferences. Our family adds a lot of superfoods to our daily green smoothies. We also enjoy hot chocolate made with raw cacao, lemon water with chia, goji berries in trail mix, and breakfast porridge (made with nuts, chia seeds, flax seeds, hemp seeds). Keep in mind that superfoods are not the only answer and becoming obsessed with any or all superfoods misses the point of whole health, true health. Our family finds superfoods to be beneficial as supplements and boosters to our diet and health habits.

Cacao (Raw Chocolate)

Cacao, yes chocolate, is one of the highest antioxidant foods on the planet. It is said to be the number one source of antioxidants, magnesium, iron, manganese, and chromium. Raw cacao improves cardiovascular health, builds strong bones, is a natural aphrodisiac, elevates your mood and energy, and increases longevity.[1] Cacao is chocolate without the cocoa butter or sugar. Most commercially available chocolate products have been so processed that they end up with very little amounts of cacao's heart-healthy flavanol antioxidants which are usually quite bitter tasting.[2] Look for products that have not undergone Dutch processing (which neutralizes cacao's natural acidity). Enjoying an ounce or two of dark chocolate that is at least 70 percent cacao a couple of times per week is actually good for our health.

Chlorella

This water-grown, micro-algae has extraordinary nutrient density. It is full of chlorophyll and contains vitamin C, all of the B vitamins, vitamin E, beta-carotene, amino acids, magnesium, iron, trace minerals, and 50 percent more protein than meat per grams of weight.[3] It also has a unique and powerful set of antioxidant properties. In addition, chlorella is a great superfood for optimizing oxygen in the blood, removing heavy metal toxins from the body, and reducing inflammation.[4]

Chia Seeds

Chia seeds are an ancient staple of the Mayans and Aztecs. The word chia means "strength" in the Mayan language. They are a superfood due to their extremely high nutrient load per calorie. They have several of the same benefits as the more well-known "super seed" flax, but unlike flax seed you don't need to grind them to reap the health benefits. Chia seeds are full of fiber, antioxidants, and protein. Chia's high calcium content delivers 18 percent of our recommended daily allowance per ounce, which is three times more than skim milk.[5] In addition, chia is full of omega-3 fatty acids, more even than salmon. It is one of the most concentrated sources of omega-3 fatty acids available. They are known to increase stamina and energy over long periods of time. Chia is a great thickener for foods—like pudding—and can be an effective egg substitute in baking for vegans or those sensitive or allergic to eggs. We throw them in our green smoothies every day to add a punch to our ninja juice.

Goji Berries

Used in traditional Chinese medicine for over five thousand years, goji berries are regarded as a longevity, strength-building, and potency food of the highest order.[6] This superfood contains eighteen amino acids, including eight essential amino acids (essential because our bodies can't make them on our own), up to twenty-one trace minerals, high amounts of antioxidants (beta-carotene, lycopene, and polyphenols), iron (more than spinach), polysaccharides (which enhance immunity), and A, B, and E vitamins. They contain more vitamin C by weight than any other food on earth.[7]

Maca

A root plant that has been a staple in the Peruvian Andes for thousands of years, this superfood is known for relieving menopause symptoms and increasing energy, endurance, fertility, strength, and libido. Dried maca powder contains more than 10 percent protein and nearly twenty amino acids, including seven essential amino acids.[8]

Hemp Seeds

Hemp seeds consist of 33 percent pure digestible protein.[9] Three tablespoons of hemp seeds provides eleven grams of protein, making these seeds a perfect food for growing children and adults looking to increase protein intake.[10] They also contain high amounts of omega-3 fatty acids, all ten essential amino acids, and are rich in phytonutrients, minerals (iron, zinc, calcium, phosphorous, magnesium) and antioxidants such as vitamin E.[11] We sprinkle these super seeds on our salads and breakfast burritos, in our smoothies, and we even eat them plain for a snack.

Spirulina

Spirulina is an algae powder that is said to be one of the most potent nutrient sources available. It is 65 percent complete protein and essential amino acids, including omega-3 fatty acids (making this supplement highly anti-inflammatory). It is rich in chlorophyll (which helps remove toxins from the blood and boost immune functioning), iron, A, B, C, and D vitamins. In addition, spirulina provides a vast array of minerals, trace elements, phytonutrients, and enzymes. Spirulina has been shown to have over twenty-six times more calcium than milk. Individuals taking any anti-coagulation medication should consult with a doctor before taking spirulina.[12]

AFA Blue-Green Algae

AFA blue-green algae is a microalgae phytoplankton best known for its ability to increase our internal production of stem cells (boosting our immune functioning significantly).[13] Unlike spirulina, this microalgae prefers fresh water. Phytoplankton have been identified as one of the first organisms to populate the earth. Some scientists predict that they have been around for nearly three billion years. They are responsible for an estimated 80 to 90 percent of the planet's overall food supply and oxygen supply. This wild-harvested food has an array of phytonutrients, a huge selection of antioxidants, B-complex vitamins, minerals (especially iron, zinc, and selenium), chlorophyll, and enzymes. It is high in easily digestible protein.[14]

Bee Products

Bee pollen is the food for young bees made by adult honeybees. It is considered one of nature's most complete foods, as it contains nearly all nutrients required by humans.[15] At approximately 40 percent protein, bee pollen is richer in protein than any animal source. Half of its protein is in a form that is ready to be directly used by the body. It contains twenty-one amino acids, more than beef, eggs, or cheese of equal weight. Bee pollen is also rich in vitamins (including B-complex) and folic acid. It boosts immune functioning, increases energy, supports the digestive and cardiovascular systems, and stimulates fertility.[16]

Now let's talk honey. Honey, in its organic, wild, raw (never heated), unfiltered state, is rich in minerals, antioxidants, probiotics, and enzymes. Raw honey has anti-viral, anti-bacterial, and anti-fungal properties, making it effective in the treatment of many types of infections. It promotes body and digestive health, is a powerful antioxidant, strengthens the immune system, and is an excellent remedy for skin wounds. Russian research indicates that wild and raw honey is a longevity superfood. If your metabolism can handle sweeteners, raw honey is the best, but consume it in moderation to avoid large blood sugar spikes. Pasteurization of honey kills all of the beneficial nutrients in the honey and is just as unhealthy as eating refined sugar.[17]

Camu Berry

Camu berries, found in Peru, Brazil, Columbia, and Venezuela, aren't usually sold in America's typical grocery stores. The camu berry fruit is the size of a lemon and bright orange in color. It is chock full of vitamin C (sixty times more per serving than an orange). One teaspoon of camu powder has 1180 percent of your recommended daily intake for vitamin C. It also contains several essential amino acids including valine. Valine prevents muscle breakdown and supports nervous system and cognitive functioning. These berries are full of antioxidants that neutralize harmful free radicals, including several different flavonoids, gallic acid, and ellagic acid. They are high in potassium. The camu berry has anti-viral properties that can help with cold sores, herpes, shingles, and the common cold. It is said to be one of the best anti-depressant, immune-building, energy-boosting, and eye-nourishing superfoods in the world.[18]

Sea Vegetables

Rich in life-giving nutrients drawn from the ocean and sun, sea vegetables help remove heavy metals, detoxify the body of radioactive iodine, provide numerous trace minerals, regulate immunity, and decrease the risk of cancer. Sea vegetables benefit the entire body and are especially beneficial for the thyroid, immune system, adrenals, and hormone function.[19] Some examples of sea vegetables include kombu, hijiki, nori, kelp, and arame. There are fantastic tasting (well, tasteless) kelp noodles available that we enjoy with stir fries and curries.

Medicinal Mushrooms

Mushrooms are said to contain some of the most potent natural medicines on the planet. Ancient Egyptians and Chinese cultures used them to promote general health and longevity. There are over 140,000 species of mushrooms on earth! Very few (about 10 percent) have been studied in science for potential health benefits. The difference between medicinal mushrooms and the button mushrooms we typically cook with (which also have their own benefits) are that medicinal mushrooms contain immune activating beta-glucans and other polysaccharides. These compounds help protect and support our immune system. Many have been proven effective in healing cancer and a variety of other ailments. Some examples of medicinal mushrooms are cordyceps, maitake, chaga, and reishi. It is important to purchase organic mushrooms (medicinal or those commonly used in cooking) because they are known to concentrate heavy metals as well as air and water pollutants.[20]

☑ LIVE IT. MODEL IT. TEACH IT.

LIVE IT.

- ☐ Don't forget to remind the brood that we should never overlook green leafy vegetables as our primary powerful superfood.
- ☐ Choose a couple of superfoods to incorporate into your diet. Rather than try to ingest every superfood every day, experiment with different varieties and assess how you feel. Allow yourself to explore one, two, or even three different superfoods to significantly enhance the punch of nutrients and antioxidants that you are getting.
- ☐ Learn more about the superfoods so you feel informed and excited about what you can gain from a few potent foods.

MODEL IT.

- ☐ Superfoods are a symbol of going above and beyond in the search for health nourishing foods. Your family will grow in their awareness of food as medicine when they see you experimenting with unconventional, yet powerful, foods.

TEACH IT.

- [ ] Share information about superfoods with your family. Inform them of the antioxidant and nutritional benefits of the various foods. Make eating these foods fun for kids by highlighting how powerful they are and how super strong they make us. They are magic foods that can make us super-hero super-eaters.

20

The Eclectic Family Table: Feeding Unique Needs

One of the biggest challenges of feeding a family well is accommodating the varying needs, preferences, and schedules of each family member. You may have a child or two with particular food sensitivities or allergies, and another that refuses to eat foods like mushrooms, onions, greens, or even any vegetables at all. On top of differing food needs and preferences, you may be dancing around multiple schedules that make it hard to sit down as a family and eat together.

Feeding Different Faces

Have you ever heard a parent say that her child refuses to eat vegetables and, therefore, just doesn't eat vegetables? Maybe you are one of those parents! This often repeated story worries me, and I have speculated on the root cause. Based on my own experience of enabling unwanted behaviors in my children, I can't help but wonder if this "no-vegetable" story is a pattern that we parents have enabled. It's true that it is impossible to force another individual to eat certain foods. I know because I have tried and failed. And I know I am not the only parent that has at times tried to just get something into my kids to keep them happy. I have observed many cases where a child refuses to eat his or her vegetables, or a healthy meal in general, and the parents simply feed them something more yummy and enticing (often more processed) to ensure that they eat something. Guilty as charged! Although seemingly harmless in the short term, the child ends up learning that he or she doesn't need to eat vegetables. Rather, in fact, he learns that if he keeps rejecting the vegetables he will eventually get something more delicious (yet less nutritious). We may actually be creating the problem ourselves.

We have developed a practice in our house to overcome this problem which seems to work fairly well. At each meal our children are given a plate with all the same nutritious foods that my husband and I have on ours (they don't get special treatment based on their preferences). If they eat everything on their plates, they qualify for a healthy snack a couple of hours later. If they do not eat everything on their plates, they can be excused without pressure, but they receive no additional food until the next meal. In addition, if there is a dessert (like fruit) involved, only those kids who clean their plates will be served. There are meals when one child or another doesn't eat his vegetables, or at times any of his meal. But usually by the next meal he is so hungry he eats everything on his plate without question. Interestingly, that plate tends to be loaded with vegetables. All of our breakfasts begin with a green smoothie, which goes down pretty fast after a skipped dinner. We find that many times the kids are motivated by the snack option and choose to eat their entire plate. By following these practices we have seen that once a child becomes used to a certain vegetable (through repetitive offerings), he grows to like it, even if he at first rejected it outright. We have learned that it is important to set boundaries around food. Cooking extra or different meals based on preferences, or providing other food options shortly after a nutritious meal, seems to simply enable poor eating habits. In our house, if a kid is not hungry enough to eat the nutrient-dense food that is on his plate, he most certainly isn't hungry enough for a dessert or treat after the meal.

One of the challenges that we have worked within our household has to do with food allergies and sensitivities. Our son has a list of allergies and sensitivities that initially made it feel tricky to feed everyone together. When we first learned of his food sensitivities, he was eighteen months old, and we were told that he should avoid corn, wheat, and dairy. I felt overwhelmed by these restrictions because those three food items, at that time in our lives, were in the majority of the food we ate. I had no idea how I was going to feed my child if I were to eliminate them, and I was daunted by the fact that I was going to have to prepare two different meals in order to accommodate his needs as well as the rest of our "needs." Fortunately, my son's sensitivities led us down a path of learning a great deal about healthy eating. We discovered that most corn, dairy, and wheat products were probably not very good for any of us to eat regularly. With some time and adaptation, our whole family eventually took most of those foods out of our diet. I fed our family a diet somewhat similar to the Paleo diet for years. Within the last six months, we found out that he also has sensitivities to eggs and almonds, which was devastating because those were common ingredients in our new style of cooking. Despite these additional challenges, we have found ways to continue eating eggs for breakfast and almonds for snacks, even though my middle child avoids them completely. We openly talk to all of our children about how some bodies do well with certain foods and some bodies don't feel good from certain foods. Our middle child is very aware and accepting that his body doesn't feel well eating certain foods, even if the rest of the family tolerates them. Because of our open conversations, he seems to take ownership of his health and what ingredients are in his food. He, without hesitation, will ask me or other adults what ingredients are in things, and he knows all of the foods that don't work for his body. He subsequently declines eating foods that have ingredients that don't agree with his body, that cause inflammation.

I have a good friend who faces a different family eating challenge. She and her husband are on a different page about what constitutes healthy eating. She has a sensitivity to wheat and believes that her whole family would benefit from eliminating wheat from their diet as well. However, her husband is not on the "no-wheat" bandwagon and not only continues to eat bread and crackers but expects to have them with meals. Because her husband chooses to eat wheat, she feels badly telling her kids that they should avoid it. Therefore, she allows the whole family to eat wheat despite what she believes to be best for them. I hear this dilemma from a lot of people, especially mothers. "I am on board, but my spouse is not. He would never go for that." Sadly, most people tend to give in or give up when they don't feel supported, encouraged, or understood by their spouse. I think they give up because lifestyle changes are hard in general, and without the support of key players the change feels hopeless and exhausting.

Similarly, I know a woman who is looking to lose weight and enhance her overall physical health. Her husband is a "meat and potatoes" guy. He needs his potato chips and burger! She feels defeated by his lack of interest in changing his eating habits, and she doesn't want to make two meals every night—one for herself and one for her husband. Consequently, they continue to eat the meals that they have eaten for years—his style, not hers. These are meals that she suspects are making them sick and overweight.

These two scenarios are certainly frustrating for the people inspired to make a healthy change. It seems that many people in this situation feel discouraged enough to give up before starting or getting very far. As with any relationship challenge that involves a difference in views or values, the solution for this scenario is not a simple one. Most of us who are in a relationship have failed at trying to change the behaviors of the other at least once, so we can all relate. The solution will be unique in each situation and will depend on the values and motivations of each individual. This topic, of course, could take up more than a few doctoral dissertations, but I would like to share a few of the insights I have had regarding how consensus might be achieved. A starting point for those of us who find ourselves in this conflict can be focusing on deep relating and connecting through safe conversation, as described in Chapter 4.

I have a personal example of how safe conversation helped my husband and me work through some food-related irritations. I have mentioned before that my husband has a nearly 100 percent full commitment to being wheat free. Choosing to eat wheat is rarely an option for him. I, on the other hand, am a little more 80/20. Most of the time I don't eat wheat, but I'm not opposed to it every now and then. There was a time when I noticed that my husband would seem to get annoyed at me when I ate wheat. He gave mostly non-verbal cues, but I could sense them, and boy did it rub me the wrong way. Eventually I brought it up with him and shared that I felt pressure from him to be absolute about wheat and that it did not feel good. We had a safe conversation listening to each other's perspectives and health goals and were amazed how simple it was to rectify our recurring conflict. My husband said that it was helpful for him to know that I didn't have the intention of never eating wheat but rather to minimize my consumption of wheat while allowing for exceptions periodically. Knowing what my eating goals were, and knowing that they were different than his, provided the insight needed to eliminate judgment. I now don't have to deal with the stink eye when I indulge in special wheat treats because he has a clearer understanding of my intentions. Safe communication may not lead to a conversion of the other's behavior, but it can at least lead to a respectful appreciation of each other's goals and values. Safe conversations about food differences are fundamental in the pursuit to hear another's perspective, needs, and feelings and together review options and solutions to ensure that everyone in the family feels heard, respected, and honored.

Another concept that I find helpful for clients is building awareness about the law of complementarity. In a nutshell, this law states that when one of us pressures another person to shift towards our perspective, the person being pressured will move further in the opposite direction. As we move away from the view of the other, he naturally begins to apply increased pressure. The more pressure that is put on us, the further our view moves in the opposing direction. The vicious cycle becomes an unproductive, conflict-ridden mess. The converse of this law is that when we lessen pressure and try to meet the other where he is (as in the example of safe conversation), when we try to understand his perspective and values, he often comes back the other direction and begins to meet us half way. The more both partners hear and validate each other the easier it is to compromise in the middle.

In some cases, I have seen that it can pay off to simply do your thing and give your partner space to do his thing. My mom began making significant changes to her diet about ten years ago. She would cook healthy foods and then be annoyed as my dad's habitual unhealthy eating patterns persisted. He continued to drink alcohol regularly and would eat processed foods and refined sugars when they were available. She resigned herself to the fact that she could not change his behaviors. She would prepare and serve healthy meals but would let him eat whatever he wanted on his own time. Once she resigned to this reality and let go of the need to change my dad, she found that he slowly began to come around on his own. Eventually, my dad just got it, and he jumped on the same bandwagon as my mom, headfirst. He is now just as committed to wellness as my mother, and they don't deviate at all on their perspective of a healthy lifestyle. My mom was wise to be patient, give him space and time, all the while holding strong to what she believed was in their best interest.

I have two friends that have done a good job of accommodating different eating in their family without adding more work, like making an extra meal. One of my friends has a six-year-old child that does not eat meat. At first this felt like an inconvenience for her, and she struggled at times knowing whether or not she should try to discourage his preference or allow him to have it. Through patience and deep listening, over time it became clear to her that he had a physical and perhaps even ethical aversion to meat that was important to him. She now supports his need to avoid meat in his diet and prepares meals that allow each family member to include or exclude meat.

Another friend has a similar meat-related family challenge. She has been a vegetarian most of her life, while her husband eats meat and is a passionate hunter. She has found a balance that works for her family. When she fixes meals, she does not include meat (to honor her values), but her husband is invited and welcome to cook and include meat in the meals for the rest of the family (to honor his values). She always offers the meat he prepares to her two small children and allows them to make decisions for themselves regarding their preferences.

Despite different food needs and preferences existing around the family table, it is important that we work together to understand each other and support each other's food related values. Turn on your deep listening, validation, and empathy skills to learn what matters most to each person, and be creative and innovative in coming up with workable solutions for everyone.

The Family Table: The Importance of Eating Together

It is not news that the average American family rarely eats together anymore. We live in a hustle and bustle world and often feel that we are just surviving as we move from one activity to another. Today, the home can be more like a hotel. People check in and check out at different parts of the day, and everyone eats different foods whenever they can. Our busy lives often make it harder to get the family together even for one meal a day. A common American household dinner consists of people eating different meals (mostly convenient, highly processed foods from a bag or box), at different times, and in front of the television, computer or smartphone, or in the car. Aside from the nutritional implications of this chaos, this lack of gathering around food may be symbolic of how poorly families are engaging with each other in general. If we can't even eat together, we are probably living separate and distracted lives on some level—resulting in ever more disconnected family relationships.

The implications of this reality are deeper than may be apparent on the surface. Research shows that families that eat together have children that do better in school, have less psychological illnesses, and are even less likely to be obese.[1] The age old saying that "the family that eats together stays together" is a reflection of this intuitive insight. Historically, American families have valued the daily ritual of sitting around a dinner table together, praying, conversing, and eating a healthy meal. Eating meals together nurtures cohesion and bonding as everyone debriefs about his/her day and talks about things that are important to him/her. The meal represents the core family values of connecting, showing up in relationship together, slowing down, listening, and truly hearing each other. Family members grow in relationship and spirit while enjoying nourishing food. In this way the dinner table can be one place where we stop and nurture our "primary foods." The traditional version of the family table going awry in our current American lifestyle is a pertinent image when reflecting on the health trends of our culture and the health of the American family.

The side effects of the evolution away from the family dinner to the scattered eating patterns of modern families, extend well beyond simply sharing fewer meals together. As highlighted throughout Part Three of this book, the foods that we now put into our bodies are derived more from manufactured processes and less from real, whole foods. As we have begun to juggle so many demands, the food industry has followed suit, offering quicker more convenient options. It is no wonder that the majority of Americans prepare convenient foods from boxes and bags or order inexpensive fast food, rather than cook fresh food at home. Not only do we feel we don't have the time to prepare whole-food meals, but we also have endless quick options available. In fact, one in four Americans reports eating at least one fast food meal every single day. In addition, the average American family now spends nearly as much money on fast food as they do on groceries. Unfortunately, when we eat out, it is difficult to eat healthy foods. Serving complete meals that cost five dollars in less than five minutes requires innovations that are not possible without preservatives, chemicals, cooking techniques, and ingredients that cannot compare to the nutritional value of home-cooked meals with real ingredients. Meals eaten outside of the home are, almost across the board, less healthy than homemade foods.

There are many reasons that eating as a family can be a challenge. My sister struggled to maintain the family meal tradition because her children were consistently hungry by five o'clock every night, but her husband didn't get home until six. So she would feed the kids something quick at five, like macaroni and cheese, chicken nuggets, or hot dogs, and then she and her husband would eat later. The two of them would sit down and eat the "real," non-processed meal that she had cooked. Never feeling okay with this situation, she kept brainstorming a solution to enable the family to eat together. She finally arrived at the answer. She now gives her kids a green smoothie at four or five so that they are able to make it to six o'clock when they can all eat together. Not only do they now all sit at the table and eat together, but her children now eat a larger variety of healthy, fresh foods because they eat what their parents are eating. This also enables them to try new vegetables and have regular conversation about healthy food. The kids *love* sitting at the table as a family and ask every night, "Can we sit all together with the family for dinner?" She has also added the post-meal healthy treat option that our family uses to incentivize the kids to finish their meal. She added a technique to our method, placing the treat in front of kids while they eat. It's rare that the kids don't attempt to eat everything on their plate in exchange for the healthy treat that awaits—literally two inches from their plates! The "family table" does not come easily for most of us, but it is well worth being creative and trying different strategies until we discover what works for each of our families.

Our family table acts as a unifier, a place of community building. Sharing a meal is an excuse to catch up, talk, and know each other more deeply. Our dinner table is a place where we not only attend to relationships but also where we talk about what is and isn't going well at work and at school. We connect with our spirits through a prayer of gratitude and by reflecting on what was meaningful in our day. We've noticed that when we eat separately we feel more removed, isolated, and estranged from each other. As outlined in Part Two, these primary food principles are truly important for our long term health, just as much as the nutritional value of the meal. From this perspective, the family table becomes a symbol of what is truly important in life and what leads to whole health. Through this symbol we can see that there is value in slowing down and prioritizing the lifestyle patterns that lead to long-term health, longevity, and happiness: focusing on both primary and secondary foods.

☑ LIVE IT. MODEL IT. TEACH IT.

LIVE IT.

- ☐ Brainstorm ways to enable the whole family to eat well. If you have picky eaters, expect that moving from eating processed foods to real foods will not likely be a seamless transition. Your family's taste buds have been trained by many years of eating a particular way. If you find that your kids don't like the new way of eating, gently encourage them to try new foods, and keep offering them healthy options. It can take up to five to seven attempts for the taste buds to get used to a new food. Be firm that what you make for a meal is the only food option, and don't offer snacks or alternatives to supplement a meal not eaten.

- ☐ Practice deep listening and safe conversations to understand each family member's food needs and come up with a plan for meals that works for everyone without turning yourself into a short order cook.

- ☐ Figure out how many nights a week it is feasible for your family to sit down at the table and eat together. I understand that for many parents this can get tricky with sport and activity schedules. My children are still too young for after-school activities, so we commit to seven days a week of eating dinner together. Perhaps for your family it will be the weekends and two days during the week. Or maybe the family meal will be breakfast before everyone runs off in his own direction. Figure out what is reasonable for your situation and make a commitment to stick to it.

- ☐ Ensure that television, phones, and computers are off limits during meal time—for parents too. Think of ways to build quality time into the structure of the meal, whether it is a prayer of gratitude at the beginning or giving all family members time and space to talk about their day, and make connecting a routine.

MODEL IT.

- ☐ Through your actions, show your family what it looks like to be clear and directed around eating healthy foods and eating together as a family. Some people may not like certain things that you cook and some kids may think that eating food around a table with everyone is a waste of time. Remember that you get to be in charge of how meals are structured and what food is served in your home. In the long run your children will discover that they can learn to like foods that are good for them.

TEACH IT.

- [ ] Talk openly to your kids about how difficult it is to feed a family with many needs. If your children are old enough, involve them in coming up with solutions that might make meal time more cohesive, efficient, and fun. Always support and choose options with which you are okay.

21

Planning and Cooking Amidst Family Mayhem

I find meal planning to be my least favorite task as a mother and keeper of the menu. As much as I love good food and can even love cooking at times, the stress of figuring out a menu and compiling a grocery list is overwhelming to me. I also work as hard as possible for meals to be simple and easy since I have busy days and very little time to "dilly dally" in the kitchen longer than is necessary. I've found that I need practical strategies to manage meal planning to avoid becoming overwhelmed and stressed. Here are some tips that I have used to make planning and cooking as easy as possible.

Web-Based Meal Planning

I find that planning ahead is critical to avoiding processed foods. When I don't have a plan, I find myself looking for a quick option, and quick options are usually not the healthiest options (going through a drive-through or popping a frozen pizza in the oven). Subscribing to eMeals, a web-based meal-planning program, has been a lifesaver in this regard. Every week now I get an email that includes seven meal suggestions based on our dietary preferences, along with the associated recipes, and a complete grocery list. There are several great meal-planning programs available on the Web—take some time to find one that might work for you. For me, the key was being provided one grocery list and menus for the whole week. eMeals has saved my sanity and has helped me cook healthy foods for my family. I am constantly making decisions throughout my day as I work, parent, and manage a house, so having my grocery list handed to me every week is like a breath of fresh air. Although I have never received a meal that we didn't enjoy, we may periodically receive one that I don't want to make or don't think my family will enjoy. In these rare cases, I simply substitute it with a meal that I know our family likes. eMeals currently offers about sixteen different food plans that you can choose from to meet your family's eating needs. We have used the Paleo meal plan and have found it closely matches our eating preferences. Other meal plans include diabetic, clean eating, gluten free, slow cooker, less than thirty minutes, vegetarian, and more, allowing you to choose the style that best suits your family. There is an inexpensive cost for the service, but I have found it to be well worth the savings in stress I used to experience trying to plan my own meals. I've also found that the meal plans have reduced trips to the grocery store significantly. Going to the store only once a week has saved me a lot of time during the week that I can now spend on other priorities.

Slow-Cooking

I love using my slow cooker. Throwing a bunch of raw food in my crock pot in the morning and having a healthy meal magically ready to go at five p.m. is a small pleasure in life that never ceases to excite me. An extra bonus of the slow cooker is that I can make enough food for multiple meals.

Double/Triple the Recipe

I thank myself a million times when I plan ahead and double or triple a menu, leaving some quick healthy meals for later in the week. Although increasing the meal size may seem like a big task at the time, reaping the benefits the following day always reminds me that it's worth it. I frequently make huge batches of soup and freeze single servings which can be heated quickly when I need an easy lunch. I also prepare large bags of our nut-based breakfast porridge in a food processor, which then lasts up to a month. I make large batches of homemade granola bars that provide quick and easy snacks for two to three weeks at a time.

Change the Way We Think About "Convenience"

When we think of convenience, most of us think of macaroni and cheese, chicken nuggets, or frozen pizza. We go right to the processed food aisle. Although processed foods are convenient and may be part of our overall survival strategy, whole food options can also be convenient. Along with the batch preparation ideas mentioned above, keeping staple "whole finger foods" in the refrigerator can be just as convenient, or even more so, than a frozen dinner. When I need a quick snack or meal for my kids, I grab simple foods like fermented pickles, lunch meat (preservative free), bell peppers, carrots, nuts, coconut flakes, nut butters with fruit or vegetables, canned beans, avocados, olives, berries, leftover green smoothies, or kale salad. Often we will make a quick burrito by throwing a mix of these items into a coconut wrap. There are many fresh food options that can be quick and convenient if we think outside of the box instead of relying on the box.

Sharing the Load

We have also found some strategies to reduce the workload on any one individual in the family. Look at your family routine to see how different family members can contribute to meal preparation. When my husband is not traveling, he prepares all the breakfasts, and I prepare all the dinners. We have also found that regularly sharing meals with other families both reduces the time any one of us spends cooking while simultaneously nurturing connection and a sense of community. I have a dear friend whose husband also travels regularly for work. We will share meals on a nearly weekly basis. We usually each contribute an easy dish or two to share and enjoy conversations about our day and how we are coping with solo parenting for the week (which naturally fills our primary food cup—and maybe wine glass!).

The bottom line is that we want to try to cook fresh foods and eat together as a family, but we need to find practical strategies that enable us to do so. Making every meal a perfectly healthy meal is probably unrealistic for most of us, but if we instead focus on each meal that we can make healthier we will find that improvements certainly are feasible. Explore different strategies and ask your friends what they do. We have learned many practical lessons by asking advice from others. As you explore you will eventually find a system that works for you. When you do find what works, share it with fellow parents. In our full and chaotic lives, most of us struggle with planning and cooking and can all learn something from each other.

☑ LIVE IT. MODEL IT. TEACH IT.

LIVE IT.

- ☐ Explore ways to plan meals so that you don't have to depend on last-minute decisions. Consider signing up for a web-based meal-planning program—like eMeals.
- ☐ Plan a couple of slow-cooker meals every week. You'll thank yourself at the end of the day when you walk in the door to a meal ready to eat.
- ☐ Double and triple recipes when you are preparing meals or snacks. Leftovers are great to duplicate meals within the week or to freeze for future quick options.
- ☐ Keep whole finger foods stocked in your home so you always have quick, healthy meals and snacks available when you are rushed.
- ☐ Connect with good friends that would enjoy sharing mealtime. Share the workload by dividing dishes to contribute to the meal.

- [ ] Ask other parents what they do to simplify meal planning and brainstorm together. Speak with older generations as many of them lived their whole lives cooking real foods, often for big families.

MODEL IT.

- [ ] Demonstrating the importance of cooking and planning meals imparts in our children an invaluable life skill. They will learn to value cooking and thoughtful meal preparation as much as you do. Whether you consistently prepare your family's food in the home with real food ingredients or rely on frozen pizza and mac and cheese, they will follow your lead. As they watch and participate in meal preparation, they will learn to appreciate the quality time, the colors, the freshness, and ultimately the process of turning fresh foods into delicious meals.

TEACH IT.

- [ ] From my perspective, it is absolutely fundamental that we teach our children how to cook. If we don't teach them, who will? It is a basic life skill that will literally set them up for healthy eating habits. Teaching meal-planning and cooking is as basic and important as teaching reading and math. I have a friend who has two "left hands" in the kitchen. She doesn't know how to cook fresh foods. She adopted this lifestyle pattern from her mother who prepared quick meals out of boxes, bags, and cans. My friend struggles with her very limited kitchen skills while wanting to eat healthy meals. Our goal is to make it as natural as possible for our children to establish lifelong healthy habits.

Conclusion

Most of our plates are full, and that isn't likely to change any time soon. Our full plates often have us racing from one place to the next or one task to the next, distracting us from what really matters. Of course, there can be value in having a full plate, but our challenge is to convert our chaotic full plate into an abundant full plate. I have written this book as a reflection of my own experience in trying to make this conversion. Sometimes it feels overwhelming, like something I will never truly achieve. Yet when I am able to slow down and focus on one small element at a time, I have found that steps forward are possible. In those moments, the little achievement feels big. And after some time the little improvements become habits and then part of who I am. After each success I find I have the energy to try one more thing. Sometimes I fall back, of course, and sometimes I move forward, but overall I feel I am moving forward. And life is truly becoming easier, I am feeling better, and I see my children avoiding illness a little more, and in general, being healthier. These small improvements motivate me to keep exploring, keep learning, and keep testing the theories. I will never truly grasp the interconnectedness of all the factors that influence our health, but baby steps in awareness lead to baby steps in lifestyle change. In this way I try to avoid thinking about perfection (which is inaccessible and debilitating) and instead stay focused on my modest objective, which is simply moving in the right direction.

Focusing on the practical solutions offered in this book can help us all convert the unhealthy elements of our full plates into health-enhancing elements of fulfilling plates. With a little attention, we are all able to take steps to enrich and deepen our connections and relationships. We all can make small steps towards being more active, sleeping better, and eating better foods. These life-enhancing changes are available to all of us. The time and attention needed to implement these changes becomes available when we begin to identify and remove the lower priority activities that are actually wasting our time.

What fills my plate is clearly going to be unique to me. And what fills your plate is unique to you. Only my own commitment to identifying what fills me and makes me whole will facilitate my own conversion. My children inspire me to model these values, as I hope they will witness and understand what it looks like to be healthy and happy. Or perhaps, even more important, is to model to them the idea that health is an ongoing journey of learning and exploring—maybe even a tool for nurturing self-awareness. As I continue to learn and re-mold the vision of what health looks like for me, I will continue to share my insights with my children. I hope to give them the tools and knowledge they need to feel empowered to make choices that lead to a long life of health, connection, satisfaction, and happiness. We have this one life to live. Let's embrace our full plate and make it a source of satisfaction, empowerment, and inspiration.

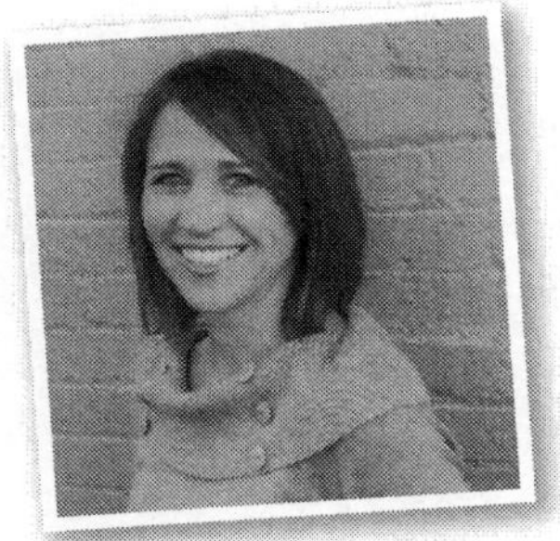

Meet the Author

Sarah Kolman lives in Lander, Wyoming, with her three young children and attentive husband—who travels regularly for work. She leads an active life raising children, managing a household, going to school, and working part-time. She holds a Bachelor of Science in Nursing and has worked in end-of-life care for over ten years. She holds a treasured Certification in Hospice and Palliative Care and has drawn great meaning and inspiration in working with this insightful and wise population. She also holds a Master of Arts in Contemplative Psychotherapy from Naropa University, where she learned the critical role of being truly present with herself and others through mindfulness practices. She is currently a student of the Institute for Integrative Nutrition®, an international nutrition program that focuses on the multi-dimensional aspects of health and wellness. She will receive a certificate as an Integrative Health Coach in the fall of 2015. Her eclectic educational, professional, and life experiences have given her rich insight into the interconnected nature of health, how to live life to the fullest, and the importance of focusing on family health. She enjoys time with her family and friends, contemplating what matters most, and learning about health and wellness.

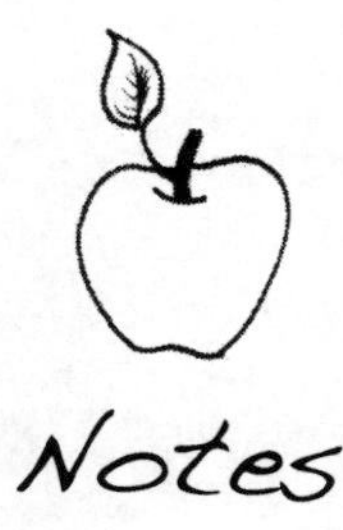

Notes

Chapter 1: Our Full Plate

1. Pam Belluck, "Children's Life Expectancy Being Cut Short by Obesity," *New York Times*, 17 March 2005, http://www.nytimescom/2005/03/17/health/17obese.html?_r=0

Chapter 2: Whole Health Philosophy

1. Joshua Rosenthal, *Integrative Nutrition: Feed Your Hunger for Health & Happiness* (New York: Integrative Nutrition Publishing, 2008). Primary and secondary food concepts developed through this reference.
2. Atul Gawande, *Being Mortal: Illness, Medicine, and What Matters in the End* (London, UK: Profile, 2014).

Chapter 3: Inflammation Affects Every Aspect of Our Health

1. Barry Sears, "Inflammation Research Foundation," DrSears.com, http://www.drsears.com/inflammation-research-foundation/.
2. David Marquis, "How Inflammation Affects Every Aspect of Your Health," Mercola.com, 7 March 2013, http://articles.mercola.com/sites/articles/achive/2013/03/07/inflammation-triggers-disease-symptoms.aspx
3. Joseph Mercola, "Doctor Says: If There's a Single Marker Lifespan, This Would Be Insulin Sensitivity," Mercola.com, 6 June 2012, http://articles.mercola.com/sites/articles/archive/2012/06/06/eft-on-chronic-inflammation.aspx
4. Christiane Northrup, "Sacred Healing with Christiane Northrup, MD, FACOG," lecture, Institute for Integrative Nutrition, New York, 9 Feb 2015.
5. Andrew Weil, "Anti-Inflammatory Health with Andrew Weil, MD," lecture, Institute for Integrative Nutrition, New York, 5 January 2015. Refeence used to develop whole paragraph.
6. Christian Nordqvist, "What Is Inflammation? What Causes Inflammation," Medical News Today, last modified 12 February 2015, http://www.medicalnewstoday.com/articles/248423.php.
7. Weil, "Anti-Inflammatory Health."

Chapter 4: Meaningful Work

1. Parker J. Palmer, *A Hidden Wholeness: The JourneyToward an Undivided Life* (SanFrancisco: Jossey-Bass, 2004).
2. Bernadetta Arena, "Oprah's Love Letter," The Quest for Life Foundation, 2 June 2011, https://qflf.wordpress.com/2011/06/02oprahs-love-letter/.
3. Brandy Bell, "The World Needs You to Come Alive," Tiny Buddha, http://tinybuddha.com/blog/the-world-needs-you-to-come-alive/, accessed 1 December 2014.
4. "Understanding the Stress Response," Harvard Health Publication, 1 Mar. 2011, http://www.health.harvard.edu/staying-healthy understanding-the-stress-response.
5. Weil, "Anti-Inflammatory Health."
6. Mayo Clinic, "Chronic Stress Puts Your Health at Risk," 11 July 2013, http://www.mayoclinic.org/healthy-living/stress-management/in-depth/stress/art-20046037.
7. Weil, "Anti-Inflammatory Health." Reference to 4-7-8 breathing content.
8. Marilena Minucci, "Self-Care with Marilena Minucci," lecture, Institute for Integrative Nutrition, New York, 3 November 2014. Reference influenced ideas in Soul-Centered Self-care section

Chapter 5: Healthy Relationships

1. Harville Hendrix, "The Nutritional Power of Relationship," lecture, Institute for Integrative Nutrition, New York, 17 November 2014.
2. *What the Bleep Do We Know?* directed by William Arntz, Betsy Chasse, and Mark Vicente (2004, Roadside Attractions), DVD.
3. Bernie Siegel, "Master the Art of Living with Bernie Siegel, MD," lecture, Institute for Integrative Nutrition, New York, 2 March 2015.
4. Joseph Mercola, "Love Really Can Cure a Broken Heart," Mercola.com. January 2010. Reference to information and research about heart and loneliness.
5. Emily Caldwell, "Loneliness, Like Chronic Stress, Taxes the Immune System," *Research and Innovation Communications*, Ohio State University, 10 January 2013. Reference for paragraph.
6. Lissa Rankin, "Mind Over Medicine with Lissa Rankin MD," lecture, Institute for Integrative Nutrition, New York, 3 November 2014.
7. Hendrix, "The Nutritional Power of Relationship."
8. Ibid.
9. Siegel, "Master the Art of Living with Bernie Siegel, MD."
10. Dan Schawbel, "Brene Brown: How Vulnerability Can Make Our Lives Better," Forbes.com, 21 Apr. 2013, http://wwforbes.com/sites/danschawbel/2013/04/21/brene-brown-how-vulnerability-can-make-our-lives-better/.

11. Brene Brown, *The Gifts of Imperfection: Let Go of Who You Think You're Supposed to Be and Embrace Who You Are* (Center City, MN: Hazelden, 2010).

12. Hendrix, "The Nutritional Power of Relationship." Reference for Improve Communication section.

Chapter 6: Regular Physical Activity and Adequate Sleep

1. "Exercise and Depression." WebMd, accessed 12 December 2014, http://www.webmd.com/depression/guide/exercise-depression.

2. Joseph Rosenthal, "The Benefits of Exercise," lecture, Institute for Integrative Nutrition, 1 December 2014. Reference to all health benefits listed in this section.

3. Peter Katzmarzyk, et al., "Sitting Time and Mortality from All Causes, Cardiovascular Disease, and Cancer," *Medicine and Science in Sports and Exercise* 41, no. 5 (2009): 998–1005, http://www.natap.org/2010/newsUpdates/SittingTimeCauses.pdf.

4. James Levine and Selene Yeager, *Move a Little, Lose a Lot: New NEAT Science Reveals How to Be Thinner, Happier, and Smarter* (New York: Crown, 2009).

5. Ibid.

6. National Sleep Foundation, "How Much Sleep Do We Really Need?" accessed 15 December 2014, http://sleepfoundation.org/how-sleep-works/how-much-sleep-do-we-really-need.

7. National Sleep Foundation, "2008 Sleep in America Poll: Summary of Findings," accessed 22 February 2015, http://sleepfoundation.org/sites/default-files/2008%20POLL%20SOF.PDF.

8. Emily Yahr, "No, You're Not Sleeping Enough, and It's a Problem: 15 Scary Facts in New NatGeo Doc," *Washington Post*, 2 December 2014. Reference to National Geographic stats in whole paragraph.

9. Kurt VonRueden, "Sleep Deprivation in the Workplace: The Hidden Side of Health and Wellness," Proceedings of ASSE Professional Development Conference, Florida, Orlando, 11 June 2014.

10. Belle B. Cooper, "10 Simple Things You Can Do Today That Will Make You Happier, Backed By Science," *Buffersocial*, Buffer.com, 6 August 2013, https://blog.bufferapp.com/10-scientifically-proven-ways-to-make-yourself-happier.

11. Camille Peri, "Coping with Excessive Sleepiness: 10 Things to Hate About Sleep Loss," WebMd, accessed 20 Dec. 2014, http://www.webmd.comsleep-disorders/excessive-sleepiness-10/10-results-sleep-loss.

12. National Sleep Foundation, "2013 Sleep in America Poll: Exercise and Sleep," 2 May 2013, http://sleepfoundation.org/sites/default/files/RPT336%20Summary%20of%20Findings%2002%2020%202013.pdf.

13. James Mass, "Consequences of Sleep Deprivation," Cornell Center for Materi als Research, 2010, http://www.ccmr.cornell.edu/ask-a-scientist/what-are-the-effects-of-sleep-deprivation.

14. National Sleep Foundation, "Sleep Deprivation Effect on the Immune System Mirrors Physical Stress," accessed 20 Dec. 2014, http://sleepfoundation.org/sleep-news/sleep-deprivation-effect-the-immune-system-mirrors-physical stress.

15. Rubin Naimen, "The Interface of Nutrition with Sleep and Dreams," lecture, Institute for Integrative Nutrition. 16 Feb 2015. Reference for slow reaction time and heightened emotions.

16. John Easton, "Fragmented Sleep Accelerates Cancer Growth," U Chicago News, 27 January 2014, http://news.uchicago.edu/article/2014/01/27/fragmented-sleep-accelerates-cancer-growth.

17. Mass, "Consequences of Sleep Deprivation."

18. National Sleep Foundation, "Sleep and Heart Disease: Are You at Risk?" accessed 12 February 2015, http://sleepfoundation.org/sleep-news/sleep-and-heart-disease-are-you-risk.

19. Mass, "Consequences of Sleep Deprivation." Reference to all statistics in para graph.

20. "Penn Medicine Researchers Show How Lost Sleep Leads to Lost Neurons," Penn Medicine, 28 March 2014, http://www.uphs.upenn.edu/news/News_Releaes/2014/03/veasey/.

21. National Sleep Foundation, "Sleep Apnea and Progressive Brain Damage," accessed 15 December 2014, http://sleepfoundation.org/sleep-news/sleep-apnea-and-progresive-brain-damage.

22. Mass, "Consequences of Sleep Deprivation." Reference to all statistics not noted in paragraph.

23. Joseph Mercola, "Your Sleeping Habits Can Have a Profound Influence on How Much You Weigh," Merola.com, 21 July 2012, http://sleepfoundation.org/sleep-news/sleep-and-heart-disease-are-you-risk.

24. VonRueden, "Sleep Deprivation in the Workplace."

25. "2013 Sleep in America Poll: Exercise and Sleep."

26. Mercola, "Doctor Says: If There's a Single Marker Lifespan, This Would Be Insulin Sensitivity." Reference to all of the sleep improvement suggestions.

27. National Sleep Foundation, "2004 Sleep in America Poll," 1 May 2004, http://sleepfoundation.org/sites/default/files/FINAL%20SOF%202004.pdf.

28. National Sleep Foundation, "Improve Your Child's School Performance with a Good Night's Sleep," accessed 20 December 2014, http://sleepfoundation.org/sleep-news/improve-your-childs-school-performance-good-nights-sleep.

29. VonRueden, "Sleep Deprivation in the Workplace."

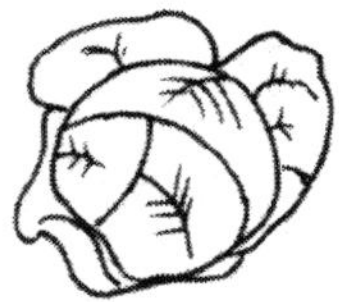

Chapter 7: Connecting to Your Spirit

1. Meredith Meinick, "Meditation Health Benefits: What the Practice Does to Your Body," *Huffpost Healthy Living,* Huffington Post, 30 April 2013, http://www.huffingtonpost.com/2013/04/30/meditation-health-benefits_n_3178731.html.

2. Susan Kuchinskas, "Meditation Heals Body and Mind," WebMD, accessed 20 December 2014, http://www.webmd.com/mental-health/features/meditation-heals-body-and-mind.

3. "Study: Meditation Actually Increases Frontal Cortex and Boosts Frontal Lobe Activity," *The Alternative Daily,* 22 April 2013, http://www.thealternativedaily.com/study-meditation-actually-increases-frontal-cortex-and-boosts-frontal lobe-activity/.

4. Julia Cameron, *The Artist's Way: A Spiritual Path to Higher Creativity* (Los Angeles: Jeremy P. Tarcher/Perigee, 1992). Reference for whole chapter.

5. Byron Katie and Stephen Mitchell, *Loving What Is: Four Questions That Can Change Your Life* (New York: Harmony, 2002). Reference for "The Work" content.

Chapter 8: Real vs. Processed Food

1. Michael Pollan, *The Omnivore's Dilemma: A Natural History of Four Meals* (New York: Penguin, 2006). Paragraph reference.

2. *Fat, Sick, & Nearly Dead,* directed by Joe Cross (2011, Joe Cross Film), DVD.

3. Joel Fuhrman, *Super Immunity: The Essential Nutrition Guide for Boosting Your Body's Defenses to Live Longer, Stronger, and Disease Free* (NewYork: HarperOne, 2011).

4. Joel Fuhrman, "The Nutrients You Need to Know with Joel Fuhrman, MD," lec ture, Institute for Integrative Nutrition, 24 November 2014.

5. Fuhrman, "The Nutrients You Need to Know."

6. Centers for Disease Control and Prevention, "Overweight and Obesity: Adult Obesity Facts," 9 September 2014, http://www.cdc.gov/obesity/data/adult.html.

7. Centers for Disease Control and Prevention, "Overweight and Obesity: Child hood Obesity Facts," 9 September 2014, http://www.cdc.gov/healthyyouth/obesity/facts.htm

8. Fuhrman, "The Nutrients You Need to Know."

9. Christiane Northrup, "Sacred Healing with Christiane Northrup, MD, FACOG," lecture, Institute for Integrative Nutrition, New York, 9 February 2015.

10. Weil, "Anti-Inflammatory Health." Reference to whole grain and water segments.

11. Kris Gunnars, "Top 10 Biggest Myths in Alternative Nutrition," Authority Nutri tion, accessed 21 February 2015, http://authoritynutrition.com/10-biggest-myths-in-alternative-nutrition/.

12. Kirtida Tandel, "Sugar Substitutes: Health Controversy over Perceived Benefits," *Journal of Pharmacology & Pharmacotherapeutics* 2, no. 4 (2011): 236–43, http://www.ncbi.nlm.nih.gov/pmc/articles/PMC3198517/.

13. "How New FDA Regulations of Trans Fat Will Make Us Healthier," *Los Angeles Daily News,* 18 November 2013, http://www.dailynews.com/health/ 20131118/how-new-fda-regulations-of-trans-fat-will-make-us-healthier.

14. Joseph Mercola, "Large Pig Study Reveals Significant Inflammatory Response to Genetically Engineered Foods," Mercola.com, 18 May 2014, http://articles.mercola.com/sites/articles/archive/2014/05/18/gmo-foods-inflammation.aspx.

15. "GMO Crops May Cause Major Environmental Risks, USDA Admits." RT, Au tonomous Nonprofit Organization, 26 February 2014, http://rt.com/usa/usda-gmo-risk-report-537/.

16. John Dill, "The Dangers of GMOs: Know the Environmental Hazards," Natural News,28 September 2010, http://www.naturalnews.com/029869_GMOs_dangers.html.

17. "GMO Facts." Non-GMO Project, accessed 10 February 2015, http://www.nongmoproject.org/learn-more/.

18. Meredith Meinick, "Proof That Fast Food Salads Are Anything But Healthy," *Huffpost Healthy Living*, Huffington Post, 29 August 2013, http://www.huffingtonpost.com/2013/08/29/fast-food-salads-not-healthier_n_3831064.html.

Chapter 9: The Top Two Eating Rules to Remember

1. Alice Walton, "How Much Sugar Are Americans Eating," Forbes, 30 August 2012, http://www.forbes.com/sites/alicegwalton/2012/08/30/how-much-sugar-are-americans-eating-infographic/. Reference for sugar statistics.

2. World Health Organization, "Obesity and Overweight," Global Strategy on Diet, PhysicalActivity and Health, World Health Organization, accessed 21 December 2014, http://www.who.int/mediacentre/factsheets/fs311/en/.

3. *Fed Up*, directed by Stephanie Soechtig (2014, Atlas Films), DVD.

4. Julie Corliss, "Eating Too Much Added Sugar Increases the Risk of Dying with Heart Disease," Harvard Health Publications, 6 February 2014, http://www.health.harvard.edu/blog/eating-too-much-added-sugar -increases-the-risk-of-dying-with-heart-disease-201402067021.

5. Jeff Volek, et al., *The Art and Science of Low Carbohydrate Living: An Expert Guide to Making the Life-saving Benefits of Carbohydrate Restriction Sustainableand Enjoyable* (Lexington, KY: Beyond Obesity, 2011).

6. Ron Rosedale, "Insulin Resistance: The Real Culprit," Drrosedale.com, 13 December 2014, http://www.drrosedale.com/resources/pdf/Insulin%20Resistance.pdf.

7. Rosedale, "Insulin Resistance."

8. Mercola, "Doctor Says: If There's a Single Marker Lifespan, This Would Be Insulin Sensitivity."

9. Stephen Sinatra, "Lower High Blood Pressure by Reducing Sugar Intake," Dr.Sinatra.com, 27 March 2014, http://www.drsinatra.com/lower-high-blood-pressure-by-reducing-sugar-intake.

10. Larry Schwartz, "9 Shocking Facts You Need to Know about Sugar," Alternet, 24 August 2014, http://www.alternet.org/food/9-shocking-facts-you-need-know-about-sugar.

11. Mercola, "Doctor Says: If There's a Single Marker Lifespan, This Would Be Insulin Sensitivity."

12. Walton, "How Much Sugar Are Americans Eating." Reference to all soda and sport drink statistics above this note in paragraph.

13. Weil, "Anti-Inflammatory Health."

14. Dain Wallis, "An Eye-Opener on Liquid Calories," Fitinafatworld.com, accessed 28 December 2014, http://fitinafatworld.com/2013/04/15/an-eye-opener-on-liquid-calories/.

15. Steve Hopkins, "Does Drinking Fruit Juice Give You High Blood Pressure? New Study Finds a Regular Morning Glass of Orange Juice Significantly Raises Health Risk," Dailymail.com, 11 October 2014, http://www.dailymail.co.uk/health/article-2789036/does-drinking-fruit-juice-high-blood-pressure-new-study-finds-regular-morningglass-orange-juice-significantly-raises-health-risk.html.

16. Zak Kardachi, "Sugar Content in Alcohol: Best and Worst." Health.com.au, accessed 12 October 2012, http://health.com.au/sugar-content-in-alcohol-best-worst/.

17. Tandel, "Sugar Substitutes."

18. Kris Gunnars, "How Sugar Hijacks Your Brain and Makes You Addicted," Authority Nutrition, accessed 27 December 2014, http://authoritynutrition.com/how-sugar-makes-you-addicted/.

19. Fuhrman, "The Nutrients You Need to Know."

20. Ibid.

21. "Phytonutrients," WebMd, accessed 20 December 2014, http://www.webmd.com/diet/phytonutrients-faq.

22. Fuhrman, "The Nutrients You Need to Know." Reference to whole paragraph.

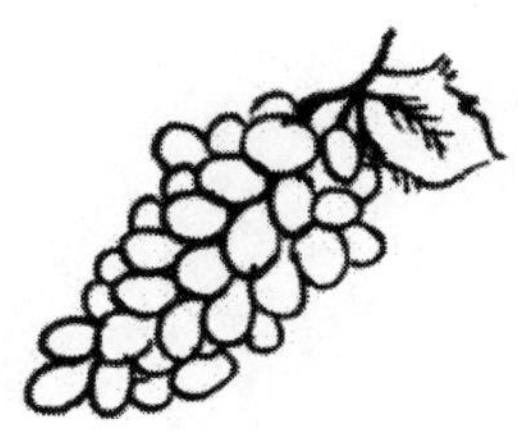

23. Victoria Boutenko, Green for Life: The Updated Classic on Green Smoothie Nutrition (Berkeley, CA: North Atlantic, 2012). Reference to whole paragraph.

24. Boutenko, Green for Life. Reference to chlorophyll information.

Chapter 10: Reading Food Labels

1. William Davis, *Wheat Belly: Lose the Wheat, Lose the Weight, and Find Your Path Back to Health* (Emmaus, PA: Rodale, 2011).

2. Weil, "Anti-Inflammatory Health."

3. David Perlmutter and Kristin Loberg, *Grain Brain: The Surprising Truth about Wheat, Carbs, Sugar—Your Brain's Silent Killers* (New York: Little, Brown and Company, 2013).

Chapter 11: How Our Microbiome Controls Our Health

1. Kathie Swift, "Heal Digestive Distress with Kathie Swift, MS, RD, LDN," lecture, Institute for Integrative Nutrition. New York, 2 February 2015.

2. Frank Lipman, "Traditional and Alternative Medicine with Frank Lipman," lecture, Institute for Integrative Nutrition, 8 December 2014.

3. "Microbiome," *Wikipedia*, last modified 13 February 2015, http://en.wikipedia.org/wiki/Microbiota.

4. Donna Gates, "Body Ecology with Donna Gates," lecture, Institute for Integrative Nutrition, New York, 2 Feb. 2015.

5. Satya Prakash, Laetitia Rodes, and Catherine Tomaro-Duchesneau, "Gut Microbiota: Next Frontier in Understanding Human Health and Development of Biotherapeutics," *Biologics* 5 (2011): 71–86.

6. Christiane Northrup, "Sacred Healing with Christiane Northrup, MD, FACOG," lecture, Institute for Integrative Nutrition, New York, 9 February 2015.

7. Natural Resources Defense Council, "Food, Farm Animals, and Drugs," accessed 30 December 2014, http://www.nrdc.org/food/saving-antibiotics.asp.

8. Weil, "Anti-Inflammatory Health" Reference to content and ideas in Microbiome Mishaps unless otherwise noted.

9. Liz Lipski, "Restore the Gut Microbiome with Liz Lipski, PhD, CCN, CNS, LDN," lecture, Institute for Integrative Nutrition, New York, 2 February 2015.

10. Centers for Disease Control and Prevention, "Show Me the Science—How to Wash Your Hands," accessed 5 Jan 2014, http://www.cdc.gov/handwashing/show-me-the-science-handwashing.html.

11. Weil, "Anti-Inflammatory Health." Reference to content and ideas in Building the Microbiome unless otherwise noted.

12. Susan Blum, "Food Is Function with Susan Blue, MD, MPH," lecture, Institute for Integrative Nutrition, New York, 9 February 2015. Reference for content in Food Allergies and Sensitivities section.

13. "Acne Bacteria Strain Linked with Healthy Skin Identified By Researchers," *Huffpost Healthy Living*, Huffington Post, 28 February 2013, http://www.huffingtonpost.com/2013/02/28/acne-bacteria-strain-healthy-skin_n_2782977.html.

14. Chris Kresser, "RHR: Naturally Get Rid of Acne By Fixing Your Gut," chriskesser.com, accessed 9 February 2015, http://chriskresser.com/naturally-get-rid-of-acne-by-fixing-your-gut.

15. Chris Kresser, "How Stress Wreaks Havoc on Your Gut—And What to Do About It," chriskresser.com, accessed 29 January 2015, http://chriskresser.com/how-stress-wreaks-havoc-on-your-gut.

16. Elsevier, "Stress Affects the Balance of Bacteria in the Gut and Immune Response," Science Daily, 22 March 2011, http://www.sciencedaily.com/releases/2011/03/110321094231.htm.

Chapter 12: Immune-Suppressed Society

1. Joel Fuhrman, *Super Immunity.*

2. Ibid.

3. Susan Blum, "Food Is Function." Reference to whole Immune Basics section.

4. Fuhrman, *Super Immunity.*

5. Mora Rodgiro, Iwata Makoto, and Andrian Ulrich, "Vitamin Effects on the Immune System: Vitamins A and D Take Center Stage," *Nature Reviews Immunology* 8, no. 9 (2008): 685–98.

6. Mineral Resource International, "Minerals and Immune Function," accessed 22 December 2014, http://www.mineralresourcesint.com/docs/news/Minerals%20and%20Immunity1.pdf?phpMyAdmin=2d45cdccf364c040257c6a71626b5a71.

7. CNCA Health, "Immune System Health and Support: The Importance of Antioxidants," accessed 18 December 2014, http://www.cncahealth.com/explore/learn/nutrition-supplements/immune-system-health-and-support-the-importance-of-antioxidants#.VPT3lI4offY.

8. Eric Metcalf, "Phytonutrients," WebMd, 29 October 2014, http://www.webmd.com/diet/phytonutrients-faq. Reference to all phytonutrient section.

9. Lipman, "Traditional and Alternative Medicine."

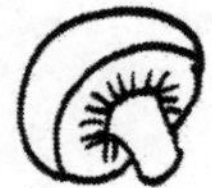

10. Christoph Thaiss, et al., "The Interplay between the Innate Immune System and the Microbiota," *Current Opinion in Immunology* 26 (2014): 41–48.

11. Kathie Swift, "Heal Digestive Distress."

12. Lipski, "Restore the Gut Microbiome."

13. "The Importance of Gut Flora For Your Immune System," Paleo Leap, accessed 28 December 2014, http://paleoleap.com/importance-gut-flora-immune-system/.

14. Fuhrman, *Super Immunity.*

Chapter 13: The Cancer Connection

1. Fuhrman, *Super Immunity.*

2. World Health Organization, "Genes and Human Disease," Genomic Re source Center, accessed 28 December 2014, http://www.who.int/genomics/public/geneticdiseases/en/index2.html.

3. Fuhrman, *Super Immunity.*

4. Ibid.

5. Michael Karin, "Cancer and Inflammation," *Nutritional Oncology,* accessed 1 January 2015, http://nutritionaloncology.org/cancerCells&Inflammation.html.

6. Charles Majors, Ben Lerner, and Ji Sayer, *The Cancer Killers: The Cause Is the Cure* (Orlando, FL: Maximized Living, 2012). Reference for whole paragraph.

7. Fuhrman, *Super Immunity.*

8. Ibid. Reference to whole chapter.

9. Ibid. Reference to whole chapter.

10. Fuhrman, "The Nutrients You Need to Know."

11. Ibid.

12. Fuhrman, *Super Immunity.* Reference to whole chapter.

13. Ibid. Reference to whole chapter.

14. Fuhrman, "The Nutrients You Need to Know." Reference to whole paragraph.

15. Fuhrman, *Super Immunity.* Reference to whole chapter.

16. Cindie Leonard, "How Do Mushrooms Prevent Breast Cancer," Livestrong.com, eHow Health, 4 August 2010, http://www.livestrong.com/article/193595-how-do-mushrooms-prevent-breast-cancer/. Reference to whole paragraph.

17. Fuhrman, *Super Immunity.* Reference to whole chapter. Reference to GBOMBS and paragraph above.

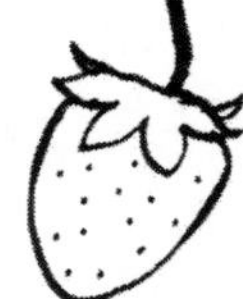

Chapter 14: Moods and Foods

1. P. Wehrewein, "Astounding Increase in Antidepressant Use by Americans," Harvard Health Publications, 20 October 2011, http://www.health.harvard.edu/blog/astounding-increase-in-antidepressant-use-by-americans-201110203624.
2. Kristin Schmidt, et al., "Prebiotic Intake Reduces the Waking Cortisol Response and Alters Emotional Bias in Healthy Volunteers," *Psychopharmacology* (2014): np.
3. Siri Carpenter, "The Gut Feeling," *American Psychological Association* 43, no. 8 (2012): 50.
4. Joseph Mercola, "What's In That? How Food Affects Your Behavior," Mercola.com, 29 July 2009, http://articles.mercola.com/sites/articles/archive/2008/07/29/what-s-in-that-how-food-affects-your-behavior.aspx.
5. Joseph Mercola, "Hike Up Your Happy Hormones with Probiotic Supplements," Mercola.com, 22 October 2011, http://articles.mercola.com/sites/articles/archive/2011/10/22/this-supplement-can-actually-make-you-happy.aspx.
6. William Duffy, *Sugar Blues* (New York: Grand Central Life & Style, 1986).
7. Blum, "Food Is Function."
8. Robynne Chutkan, "Could Leaky Gut Be What's Troubling You?," The Dr. Oz Show, Harpo, 20 February 2013, http://www.doctoroz.com/article/could-leaky-gut-be-troubling-you.
9. Joseph Mercola, "The Depressing Truth about Vitamin D Deficiency," Mercola.com, 30 December 2006, http://articles.mercola.com/sites/articles/archive/2006/12/30/the-depressing-truth-about-vitamin-d-deficiency.aspx
10. Weil, Andrew, "Embracing Your Mood: Achieving Emotional Sea Level," *Self Healing*, Feb. 2014, 4–5.
11. Weil, "Embracing Your Mood."
12. Angela Haupt, "Food and Mood: 6 Ways Your Diet Affects How You Feel," *U.S. News and World Report*, 31 August 2011.
13. Willow Lawson, "Omega-3s For Boosting Mood," *Psychology Today*, 16 August 2007.
14. Chris Iliades, "Foods That Fight Depression," Everyday Health, accessed 27 Dec. 2014, http://www.everydayhealth.com/depression-pictures/8-foods-that-fight-depression.aspx.
15. Weil, "Embracing Your Mood."

Chapter 15: Influencing Inflammation With Food

1. Weil, "Anti-Inflammatory Health."
2. Barry Sears, "The Wellness Zone with Barry Sears, PhD," lecture, Institute for Integrative Nutrition," 5 January 2015. Reference to whole paragraph.
3. Ibid., Reference to whole paragraph.

4. Ibid., Reference to whole paragraph. 5. Ibid., Reference to whole paragraph.

6. Andrew Weil, "Anti-Inflammatory Diet & Pyramid," Weil Lifestyle, accessed 20 December 2014, http://www.drweil.com/drw/u/PAG00361/anti-inflammatory-food-pyramid.html. Reference to proinflammatory graph and anti--inflammatory graph unless otherwise noted.

7. "Top 10 Anti-Inflammatory Foods You've Got to Know," The Conscious Life, accessed 20 December 2014, http://theconsciouslife.com/top-10-anti-inflammatory-foods.htm.

8. Ibid.

9. Amanda MacMillan, "14 Foods That Fight Inflammation," Health, accessed 20 December 2014, http://www.health.com/health/gallery/0,,20705881,00.html.

10. Ibid.

11. bid.

12. Ibid. Reference to whole nut and seeds section.

13. Weil, "Anti-Inflammatory Health."

14. "Avocados," *The World's Healthies Foods.* George Mateljan Foundation, accessed 20 December 2014, http://www.whfoods.com/genpage.php?tname=foodspice&dbid=5.

15. MacMillan, "14 Foods That Fight Inflammation."

16. Ibid.

17. Ibid.

18. Ibid.

19. Frank Lipman, "The Basics on Grass Fed Meat." Dr. Frank Lipman, Mar 2014, http://www.drfranklipman.com/the-basics-on-grass-fed-meat/.

20. MacMillan, "14 Foods That Fight Inflammation."

21. Ibid.

22. Sears, "The Wellness Zone with Barry Sears, PhD."

23 Weil, "Anti-Inflammatory Diet & Pyramid." Reference to proinflammatory graph and antiinflammatory graph unless otherwise noted.

24. "Top 10 Anti-Inflammatory Foods You've Got to Know."

25. Weil, "Anti-Inflammatory Diet & Pyramid." Reference to proinflammatory graph and antiinflammatory graph unless otherwise noted.

26. "Top 10 Anti-Inflammatory Foods You've Got to Know."

27. Sears, "The Wellness Zone with Barry Sears, PhD." Reference to whole paragraph and table.

Chapter 16: Organic, Grass-Fed, and Other Food Labels

1. FAO Inter-Departmental Working Group on Organic Agriculture, "Why Is Organic Food More Expensive Than Conventional Food?" *Organic Agriculture*, accessed 28 December 2014, http://www.fao.org/organicag/oa-faq/oa-faq5/en/. Reference to content in whole paragraph.
2. "What Does Organic Mean?" Organic.org, accessed 28 December 2014, http://www.organic.org/home/faq.
3. Miles McEvoy, "Organic 101: What the USDA Organic Label Means," United States Department of Agriculture, 22 March 2012, http://blogs.usda.gov/2012/03/22/organic-101-what-the-usda-organic-label-means/.
4. Dominque Mosbergen, "Organic Food Has More Antioxidants, Less Pesticide Residue: Study," *Huffpost Green*. Huffington Post, 12 July 2012, http://www.huffingtonpost.com/2014/07/12/organic-food-study_n_5579174.html.
5 Alan Henry, "What Does Organic Really Mean, and Is It Worth My Money?" *Lifehacker*, 10 September 2012, http://lifehacker.com/5941881/what-does-organic-really-mean-and-should-i-buy-it.
Health benefit section of book was significantly influenced by this article.
6 Lawrence Robinson, et al., "Are Organic Foods Right for You: Under standing the Benefits of Organic Foods and the Risk of GMOs and Pesticides," Helpguide.org, December 2014, http://www.helpguide.org/articles/healthy-eating/organic-foods.htm.
7. William Hudson, "Should You Buy Organic? Study Complicates Decision?" CNN, 4 September 2012. Reference for quote and stats in whole paragraph.
8. Mosbergen, "Organic Food Has More Antioxidants, Less Pesticide Residue."
9. Swift, "Heal Digestive Distress."
10. David Bronner, "Herbicide and Insecticide Use on GMO Crops Skyrocketing While Pro-GMO Media Run Interference," *Huffpost Green*, Huffington Post, 15 November 2014, http://www.huffingtonpost.com/david-bronner/herbicide-insecticide-use_b_5791304.html.
11. National Resources Management and Environmental Department, "Organic Agriculture and Climate Change," Food and Agriculture Organization of the United Nations, FAO Corporate Document Repository.
12. "Health Benefits of Organic Agriculture," Beyond Pesticides, accessed 2 January 2015, http://www.beyondpesticides.org/organicfood/health/.
13. Stephan Rechtschaffen, "The Future of Food Allergies with Stepha Rechtschaffen, MD," lecture, Institute for Integrative Nutrition, 26 January 2015.
14. Environmental Working Group, "All 48 Fruits and Vegetables with Pesticide Residue Data," April 2014, http://www.ewg.org/foodnews/list.php.
15. Robinson et al., "Are Organic Foods Right for You."

16. Mayo Clinic, "Organic Foods: Are They Safer? More Nutritious?" accessed 28 December 2014, http://www.mayoclinic.org/healthy-living/nutrition-and-healthy-eating/in-depth/organic-food/art-20043880. Reference for content in whole paragraph.

17. Human Society of the United States, "How to Read Egg Carton Labels: A Brief Guide to Labels and Animal Welfare," 3 July 2014, http://www.humanesociety.org/issues/confinement_farm/facts/guide_egg_labels.html.

18. Robinson, et al., "Are Organic Foods Right for You."

19. Ibid.

20. Ibid.

21. "How to Read Egg Carton Labels."

22. Ibid.

23. Ibid.

24. "Corn, Cows, Feedlots & Your Health," Onlygrassfed.com, accessed 29 December 2014, http://onlygrassfed.com/pasture-vs-feedlot.html.

25. Joseph Mercola, "Why Grassfed Animal Products Are Better for You," Mercola.com, accessed 30 December 2014, http://www.mercola.com/beef/health_benefits.htm.

26. "Corn, Cows, Feedlots & Your Health." Reference to whole paragraph.

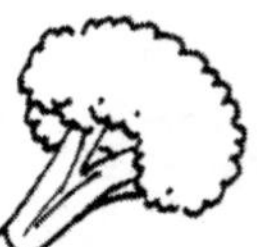

Chapter 17: Milk, Does It Do a Body Good?

1. "Should Adult Humans Drink Milk? Study of Neolithic Farmers May Have the Answer," Ancient Origins, 30 August 2013, http://www.ancient-origins.net/news-general/should-humans-drink-cow-s-milk-new-study-neolithic-farmers-may-have-answer-00787.

2. Joseph Mercola, "Don't Drink Your Milk," Mercola.com, accessed 27 December 2014, http://www.mercola.com/article/milk/no-milk.htm. Reference for information in whole paragraph.

3. Ibid. Reference for information in whole paragraph.

4. Ibid. Reference for Pasteurization and Processing section

5. Walter Willett, "Optimize Your Diet with Walter Willett, MD, DrPH," lecture, Institute for Integrative Nutrition, 16 February 2015.

6. Barnard, "Increased Calcium Intake Does Not Reduce Bone Fractures or Osteoporosis," The Physicians Committee, 27 May 2011, http://www.pcrm.org/media/blog/may2011/increased-calcium-intake-does-not-reduce-bone.

7. Joshua Rosenthal, "Bone Health," lecture, Institute for Integrative Nutrition, 8 December 2014. Reference to information in Milk, Calcium, and Bones section, unless otherwise noted.

8. Mercola, "Don't Drink Your Milk."

9. Rosenthal, "Bone Health."

Chapter 18: What's the Deal With Wheat?

1. Rachel Begun, "Gluten-Free Living with Rachel Begun, MS, RD," lecture, Institute for Integrative Nutrition, 26 January 2015. Reference to whole paragraph.
2. William Davis, *Wheat Belly.*
3. Ibid
4. Perlmutter and Loberg, *Grain Brain.*
5. Davis, *Wheat Belly.*
6. Weil, "Anti-Inflammatory Diet & Pyramid."
7. Davis, *Wheat Belly.* Reference to whole paragraph.

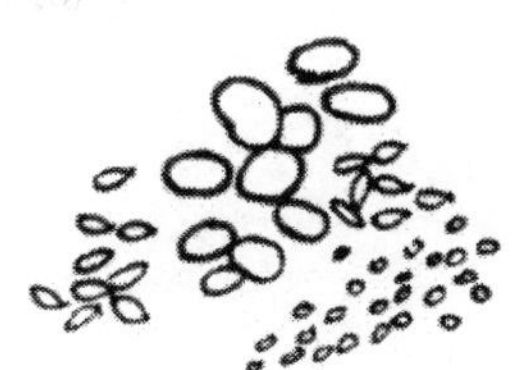

Chapter 19: Super Health With Superfoods

1. David Wolfe, "Raw Vitality with David Wolfe," lecture, Institute for Integrative Nutrition, 17 November 2014.
2. Weil, "Anti-Inflammatory Diet & Pyramid."
3. Willow Tohl, "Chlorella 101: What You Need to Know about This Nourishing Superfood," *Natural News,* 30 May 2012, http://www.naturalnews.com/036086_chlorella_superfood_algae.html.
4. Wolfe, "Raw Vitality with David Wolfe."
5. Terri Coles, "Chia Seed Benefits: 10 Reasons to Add Chia To Your Diet," *Huffpost,* Huffington Post, 26 January 2015, http://www.huffingtonpost.ca/2013/06/03/chia-seed-benefits-_n_3379831.html.
6. Wolfe, "Raw Vitality with David Wolfe."
7. David Jockers, "The Superfood Power of Goji Berries," *Natural News,* 29 May 2012, http://www.naturalnews.com/036003_goji_berries_superfood_nutrients.html.
8. Wolfe, "Raw Vitality with David Wolfe."
9. Ibid.
10. "Benefits of Hemp Seeds: 8 Reasons You Should Eat Them," *Healthy Body Now,* accessed 20 December 2014, http://healthybodynow.net/benefits-of-hemp-seeds-8-reasons-to-eat-them/.
11. Wolfe, "Raw Vitality with David Wolfe."
12. Ibid. Reference to whole paragraph.
13. Ibid.
14. Marita Mason, "AFA Super Blue-Green Algae Primordial Food from Klamath Lake Oregon," Stem Cell Nutrition, accessed 28 December 2014, http://www.stemcellnutrition.net/afa-super-blue-green-algae.
15. Wolfe, "Raw Vitality with David Wolfe."

16. Joseph Mercola, "The Use of Bee Pollen as a Superfood," Mercola.com, 17 November 2009, http://www.mercola.com/article/diet/bee_pollen.htm.

17. Wolfe, "Raw Vitality with David Wolfe."

18. Terri Coles, "Camu Camu Benefits: 11 Things You Need to Know About the Fruit," *Huffpost Living*, Huffington Post, 23 January 2014, http://www.huffingtonpost.ca/2013/07/25/camu-camu-benefits-_n_3644392.html.

19. Wolfe, "Raw Vitality with David Wolfe."

20. Heidi Georg, "Medicinal Mushrooms: The Ancient Superfood," Breaking Muscle, accessed 5 February 2015, http://breakingmuscle.com/nutrition/medicinal-mushrooms-the-ancient-superfood. Reference to the whole paragraph.

Chapter 20: The Eclectic Family Table: Feeding Unique Needs

1. Cody C. Delistraty, "The Importance of Eating Together," *The Atlantic*, 18 July 2014, http://www.theatlantic.com/health/archive/2014/07/the-importance-of-eating-together/374256/.

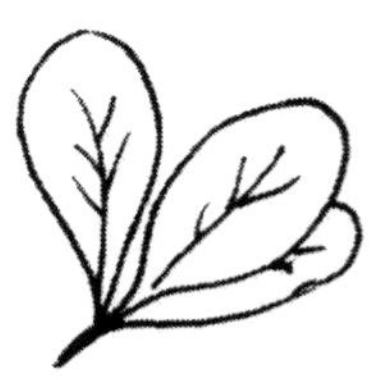

Made in the USA
Middletown, DE
01 December 2016